Other monographs in the series, Major Problems in Clinical Pediatrics:

Altman and Schwartz: *Malignant Diseases of Infancy, Childhood and Adolescence*—1978

Avery, Fletcher and Williams: *The Lung and Its Disorders in the Newborn Infant*—Fourth Edition, 1981

Bell and McCormick: *Increased Intracranial Pressure in Children*—Second Edition, 1978

Bell and McCormick: *Neurologic Infections in Children*—Second Edition, 1981

Brewer: *Juvenile Rheumatoid Arthritis*—1970

Cornblath and Schwartz: *Disorders of Carbohydrate Metabolism in Infancy*—Second Edition, 1976

Dubowitz: *Muscle Disorders in Childhood*—1978

Gryboski: *Gastrointestinal Problems in the Infant*—1975

Hanshaw and Dudgeon: *Viral Diseases of the Fetus and Newborn*—1978

Harrison and Harrison: *Disorders of Calcium and Phosphate Metabolism in Childhood and Adolescence*—1979

Lubchenco: *The High Risk Infant*—1976

Markowitz and Gordis: *Rheumatic Fever*—Second Edition, 1972

Oski and Naiman: *Hematologic Problems in the Newborn*—Second Edition, 1972

Rowe, Freedom and Mehrizi: *The Neonate with Congenital Heart Disease*—Second Edition, 1980

Royer, et al: *Pediatric Nephrology*—1974

Scriver and Rosenberg: *Amino Acid Metabolism and Its Disorders*—1973

Smith: *Recognizable Patterns of Human Malformation*—Second Edition, 1976

Smith: *Growth and Its Disorders*—1977

Solomon and Esterly: *Neonatal Dermatology*—1973

Solomon, Esterly and Loeffel: *Adolescent Dermatology*—1978

Forthcoming Monographs

Belman and Kaplan: *Urologic Problems in Pediatrics*

Bluestone and Klein: *Otitis Media in Infants and Children*

Drash: *Juvenile Diabetes*

Glader: *Anemias in Children*

Griffin: *Children's Orthopedics*

Ingelfinger: *Pediatric Hypertension*

Kerns: *Child Abuse and Neglect*

Volpe: *Neurology of the Newborn*

RECOGNIZABLE PATTERNS OF HUMAN DEFORMATION

Identification and Management of Mechanical Effects on Morphogenesis

by
David W. Smith, M.D.
Dysmorphology Unit
Department of Pediatrics
University of Washington Medical School
Seattle, Washington

Volume XXI in the Series
MAJOR PROBLEMS IN
CLINICAL PEDIATRICS

ALEXANDER J. SCHAFFER
Consulting Editor
MILTON MARKOWITZ
Associate Consulting Editor

W. B. Saunders Company, Philadelphia, London, Toronto, Sydney 1981

W. B. Saunders Company: West Washington Square
Philadelphia, Pa. 19105

1 St. Anne's Road
Eastbourne, East Sussex BN21 3UN, England

1 Goldthorne Avenue
Toronto, Ontario M8Z 5T9, Canada

9 Waltham Street
Artarmon, N.S.W. 2064, Australia

Recognizable Patterns of Human Deformation ISBN 0-7216-8401-7

 Press of W. B. Saunders Company. Library of Congress catalog card number 80-51325.

Last digit is the print number: 9 8 7 6 5 4 3 2 1

Dedication

To the Dysmorphology Fellows,
the life blood of the Dysmorphology Unit,

and

To Eleanor, Jane, and Anne,
My mother and two sisters,
who have been a source of inspiration and support.

Foreword

This is the author's third book in the monograph series, the David W. Smith trilogy on normal and abnormal physical growth and development. Doctor Smith is already very well known for his first volume, *Recognizable Patterns of Human Malformation,* published in 1970 and now in its second edition. That volume continues to be extraordinarily useful and it has become the standard pediatric reference for dysmorphology. His second book, *Growth and Its Disorders,* published in 1977, covered that important subject thoroughly and concisely.

In this book, Doctor Smith discusses yet another group of deviations from normal, those due to mechanical forces in the intrauterine environment. These are defined as *deformations* caused by external factors and are distinct from malformations due to intrinsic abnormalities of the fetus. Many physicians have not given enough thought to this distinction, but, as Doctor Smith points out, it is of considerable practical importance for advising parents about prognosis and recurrence risk, since these are generally more favorable for deformations than for malformations.

The material on deformations is presented in the usual Smith style, a well illustrated compendium, clearly and concisely written and full of usable information.

MILTON MARKOWITZ

Acknowledgments

It was in February, 1975, at an international meeting on nomenclature for birth defects, that I first heard Peter Dunn, M.D., of Bristol, England, give his impassioned plea for a clear distinction between defects due to mechanical constraint forces (deformation) as contrasted to those due to poor formation (malformation). His recommendation was accepted forthwith. Since that time I have been ever more impressed by the importance, relevance, and magnitude of this deformational category of birth defects. Hence, I acknowledge Peter Dunn as the individual who set me forth on the pathway that culminated in this book.

I wish to also express my gratitude for the knowledge and materials gained from Professor Gian Töndury, retired Professor of Anatomy at the University of Zürich, which have been of great value in this treatise.

Fellows in training have been the life blood of the Dysmorphology Unit, as mentioned in the dedication. Those involved directly in the development of this book have been Sterling Clarren, M.D., and John Graham, M.D. Visitors to the Dysmorphology Unit who have made valuable contributions and critiques include Dr. Roy Carlson (Portland, Oregon), Dr. Manuel Hernandez (Madrid), Dr. Pedro Hernandez (Caracas), and Dr. Steven Simons (Omaha). Dr. Manuel Hernandez kindly translated the excellent historical perspective on mechanically induced structural defects in the Italian book by C. Taruffi: *Storia della teratologia,* eight volumes, Bologna, Regia Tipografia, 1881. The pediatric orthopedic critique of Dr. Lynn Staheli (Children's Orthopedic Hospital) and the obstetrical review of the book by Dr. Larry Karp (Swedish Hospital) were extremely helpful. Becky Bunn, R.N., and the other nursing staff of the newborn nursery of the Group Health Cooperative have been most helpful in alerting us to examples of deformations among newly born babies.

Ms. Mary Ann Sedgwick Harvey, research associate and "Jill of all trades" for the Dysmorphology Unit deserves full credit for most of the photography as well as for invaluable editorial assistance. The majority of photographs were made from color slides, which limits the sharpness of black and white copies. We appreciate the able assistance of the photography group of the Health Sciences Learning Resource Center at the University of Washington in solving this problem.

The great majority of medical illustrations were prepared by Ms. Phyllis Wood of the Health Sciences Learning Resource Center, who has been a godsend in the development of this book and others from the Dysmorphology Unit.

Lyle M. Harrah, the Dysmorphology Research Librarian, has, despite her youthful 84 years, been of inestimable value. In addition to the references that are quoted, she provided a host of background literature that is not quoted. Mrs. Carole Stock also assisted in locating relevant photographs.

Ms. Judith Williams not only showed great expertise in the secretarial development of this book but contributed important editorial critiques as well. Her assistance is greatly appreciated.

Ann Smith, my wife, deserves a major credit for this book as well as others from the Dysmorphology Unit. She provides the type of general and background support and encouragement that allows such undertakings to evolve and occur without undue tribulation.

DAVID SMITH

Contents

Chapter One

INTRODUCTION

"Action is equal to reaction; and in the contrary direction."

Mechanical forces play an important role in both normal and abnormal morphogenesis. Anomalies that represent the normal response of a tissue to unusual mechanical forces are termed *deformations,* in contrast to *malformations,* which denote a primary problem in the morphogenesis of a tissue, and *disruptions,* which represent the breakdown of a previously normal tissue. There are predominantly two types of deformation problems: those in which the causative forces were due to an intrinsic problem of the fetus,* such as a malformation, and those in which the deformation was produced by mechanical forces that were extrinsic to an otherwise normal fetus.

Some of the intrinsic deformations secondary to a malformation are considered in Chapter 4. This text is primarily concerned with *extrinsic deformations* produced by constraint in utero of an otherwise normal fetus. Extrinsic forces may cause a single localized deformation, such as a deformed foot, or they may cause a deformation sequence. A deformation sequence refers to the manifold molding effects of a given deforming situation. A good example is the oligohydramnios sequence, in which oligohydramnios is responsible for a number of deformations. The single deformations are presented in atlas form along with the deformation sequences. The major cause of such deformations is uterine constraint of the rapidly growing malleable fetus in late gestation as the fetus tends to outgrow the uterus. Most of the molded deformations have an excellent prognosis, once the fetus is released from the constraining environment. However, some of them merit treatment, and this usually involves the use of gentle mechanical forces to attempt to *reshape* the anomaly to a more normal form.

A clear distinction between deformation and malformation is critical to providing the parents with a clear understanding of the problem and its prognosis, management, and recurrence risk. In general, the prognosis is *much* more favorable if the problem is deformation rather than malformation. The collective frequency of extrinsic deformations of late fetal origin, such as those set forth in Chapter Two, is about 2 per cent of liveborn babies. Hence, this text deals with common problems.

A broader clinical approach toward the problems of deformation is presented in Chapter Three, and the basic principles of biomechanics plus the role of mechanical factors in the normal as well as abnormal morphogenesis of particular tissues are set forth in Chapter Four.

*The embryo and fetus are collectively referred to as the fetus in this text. Fetus in Latin basically means "the young one."

REFERENCE

1. Dunn, P.M.: The influence of the intrauterine environment in the causation of congenital postural deformities, with special reference to congenital dislocation of the hip. (Thesis for M. D. degree.) University of Cambridge, 1969.

Chapter Two

PATTERNS OF DEFORMATION

1.0 JOINT CONTRACTURE, ESPECIALLY OF THE FOOT

GENERAL. Any cause that gives rise to prolonged immobilization of a joint tends to give rise to joint fixation with contracture. This can result from immobilization due to external constraint, from intrinsic neuromuscular problems, or from defects in the formation of the joint and/or its connective tissue, as summarized in Figure 2–1. When the problem is the result of external constraint the position of a given joint reflects the nature of the forces that resulted in the deformation. The most common region affected is the foot, though fixations of other joints may also occur. When there are fixations of multiple joints the term arthrogryposis is utilized. This term designates a category and *not* a diagnosis.

According to Ruth Wynn-Davies,[1] congenital malposition of the foot, often loosely referred to as clubfoot, occurs with a frequency of about 4 per 1000 births. Probably more than half of these represent deformations due to external constraint in utero. The prognosis is much better for this constraint category than for any of the other causes of joint contracture.

Evaluation of the foot includes determining the full range of its mobility. Roentgenograms are of little value in early infancy because the bones are not sufficiently ossified to allow for a relevant assessment. Among the associated anomalies that tend to occur with *postural* equinovarus or calcaneovalgus types of foot deformities are joint

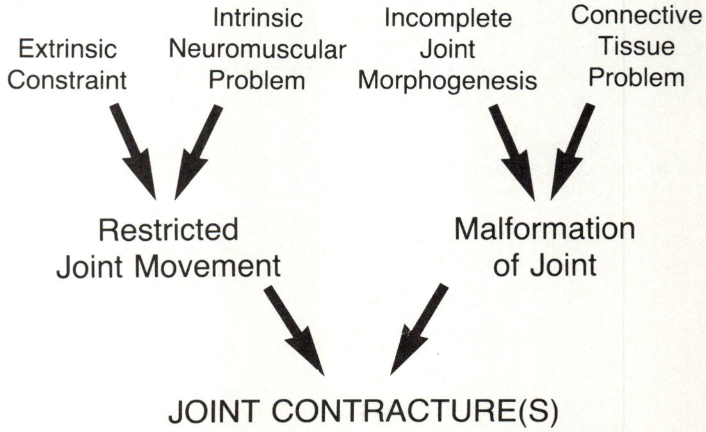

Figure 2–1. Joint contracture at birth may be the consequence of a number of modes of developmental pathology, of which in-utero constraint is the most common.

Table 2–1. Methods of Management for Foot Contracture

METHOD	COMMENT
Manual stretching, toward normal form	Performed at each feeding and diaper change
Adhesive taping, toward normal form	This method is gaining in popularity. Use tincture of benzoin to protect the skin
Splinting	Devices such as the Denis-Browne splint and reversed-last shoes may be utilized, especially at night, to maintain desired position
Plaster cast	Though casting may be utilized to correct position, it is best used to maintain an improved form which has been achieved by manipulation, taping, and/or surgery
Surgery	If more conservative measures have not resulted in improvement of foot position during early infancy, surgery merits consideration. The present tendency is to operate earlier on resistant cases, including those that are secondary to a neurological problem

laxity (10 per cent) and inguinal hernia (7 per cent). These findings suggest that minor connective tissue problems may enhance the liability to positional deformation of the foot. The postural deformities that have had their onset in utero may be perpetuated by particular sleeping postures in early infancy. Hence, consideration of sleeping posture and whether it is or is not augmenting the deformation may be an important part of the evaluation.

A number of modes of management have been utilized in attempts to restore the foot to its usual position.[2] These are summarized in Table 2–1. Alteration of sleeping posture is another consideration. Each type of foot contracture should be considered individually, as to both prognosis and management. For example, the prognosis for calcaneovalgus with manipulative stretching alone is usually excellent, whereas about half of the cases of equinovarus contracture resist correction by conservative measures. This is one of the many reasons why I believe the term "clubfoot" should be eliminated.

REFERENCES

1. Wynne-Davies, R.: Family studies and aetiology of club foot. J. Med. Genet. *2*:227, 1965.
2. Lloyd-Roberts, G.C.: Orthopaedics in Infancy and Childhood. New York, Appleton-Century-Crofts, 1971.
3. Chung, C.S., Nemechek, R.W., Larson, I.J., and Ching, G.H.S.: Genetic and epidemiological studies of clubfoot in Hawaii. Hum. Hered. *19*:321, 1969.
4. Hansen, S.T.: The child's foot: evaluation and treatment. Independent Learning Program, School of Medicine, University of Washington, 1978.

1.1 CALCANEOVALGUS

(Dorsiflexed Foot)

GENESIS. This deformity, which has a frequency of 1/1000,[1] is most commonly the result of uterine constraint having forced the foot into a dorsiflexed position against the lower leg. It is especially common with extended legs following prolonged breech position. Partly for this reason, it has a non-random association with dislocation of the hip. Dislocation of the hip, which is found in 5 per cent of patients with calcaneovalgus,[1] obviously merits high risk consideration in any newborn with this foot deformity. Calcaneovalgus is more common in firstborn infants and about four times more common in females than in males.[1] This latter observation may relate to the greater degree of joint laxity in females than in males. In keeping with this hypothesis, there is an increased frequency (10 per cent) of joint laxity in first degree relatives of children with this anomaly.[1]

FEATURES. The foot is dorsiflexed toward the fibular side of the lower leg. This has often resulted in a posterior displacement of the lateral malleolus in association with pressure-induced deficiency of subcutaneous adipose tissue at the presumed site of folding compression and in unusual skin creases at the site of the dorsiflexion of the foot at the ankle. The heel may be in valgus position relative to the ankle but the bones of the foot itself are usually in normal alignment.

MANAGEMENT, PROGNOSIS, AND COUNSEL. The foot is most commonly flexible. With no therapy or with passive stretching toward a normal position, there is usually a rapid return toward normal form. If the improvement is not rapid, then taping may be utilized. If the situation has not resolved by four to six months, the use of night braces and/or casting merits consideration. The frequency of this deformity by history in first degree relatives (parents and siblings) is 2.6 per cent.[1]

DIFFERENTIAL DIAGNOSIS. The deformity may be secondary to neurological deficiency, as in meningomyelocele.

Congenital vertical talus is a rather rare inherited deformity that may yield a foot in similar position to calcaneovalgus at birth. There is muscle atrophy and the foot is stiff. The calcaneus is displaced posteriorly and the talus displaced downward, yielding a rocker-bottom foot. These are difficult to treat, and it usually requires early casting and early surgery to achieve a functional foot.

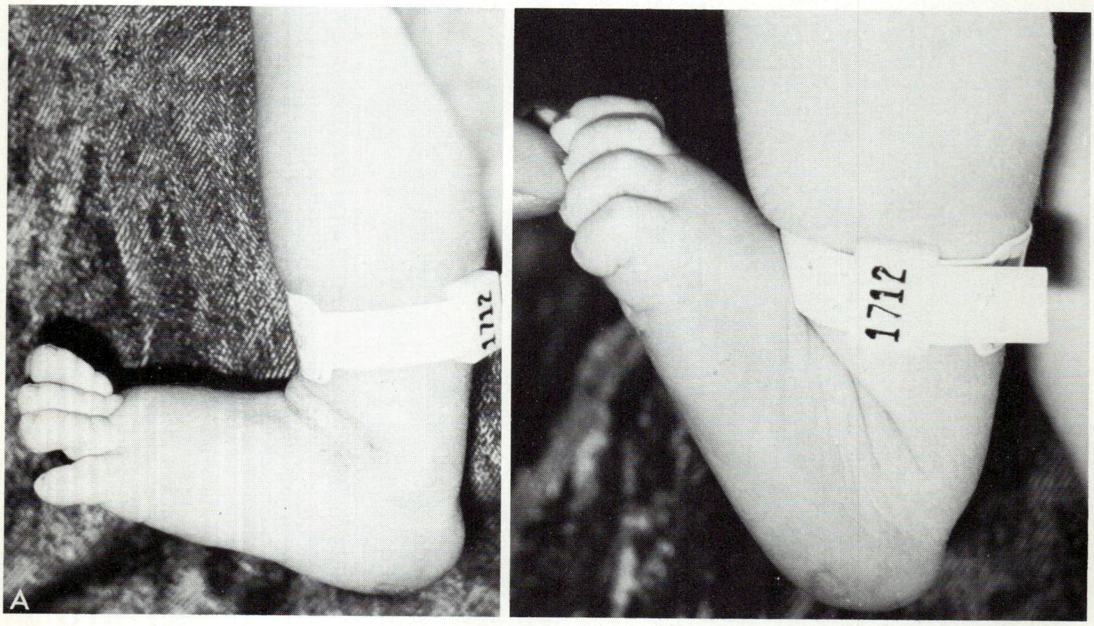

Figure 2–2. *A*, Gentle pressure (right) re-creates the presumed in-utero position of this foot which engendered the calcaneovalgus positioning.

Illustration continued on opposite page

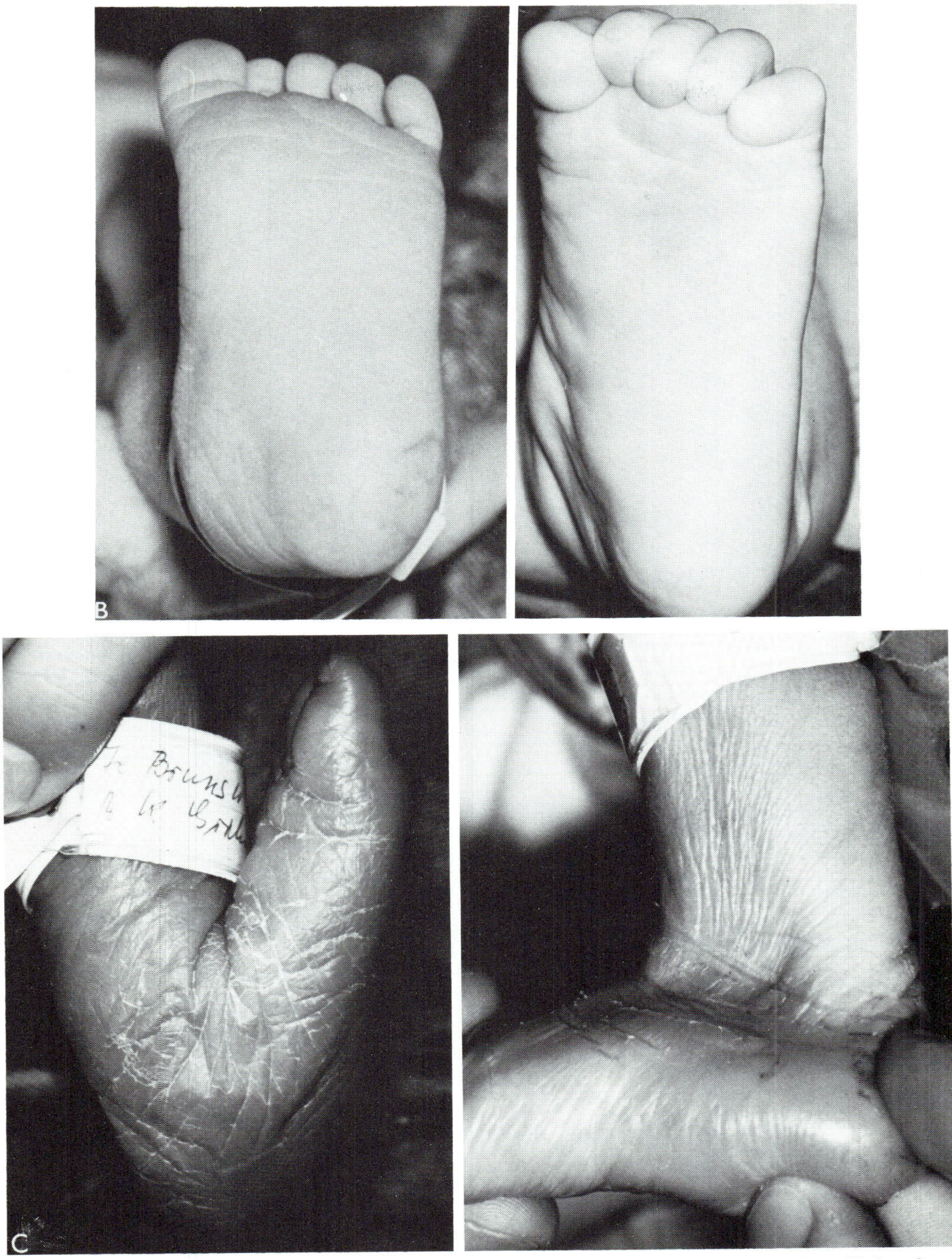

Figure 2–2 *Continued.* *B,* Left, the valgus deviation of the heel is evident in this view. Right, the same foot with simple manipulation at 12 weeks. *C,* Left, medial view of a severely molded calcaneovalgus foot. With ventriflexion of the foot, the lateral view shows the creases, the shallow sulcus, and the posterior displacement of the lateral malleolus and valgus position of the heel which are the consequences of long-term dorsilateral positioning of the foot in utero.

Illustration continued on following page

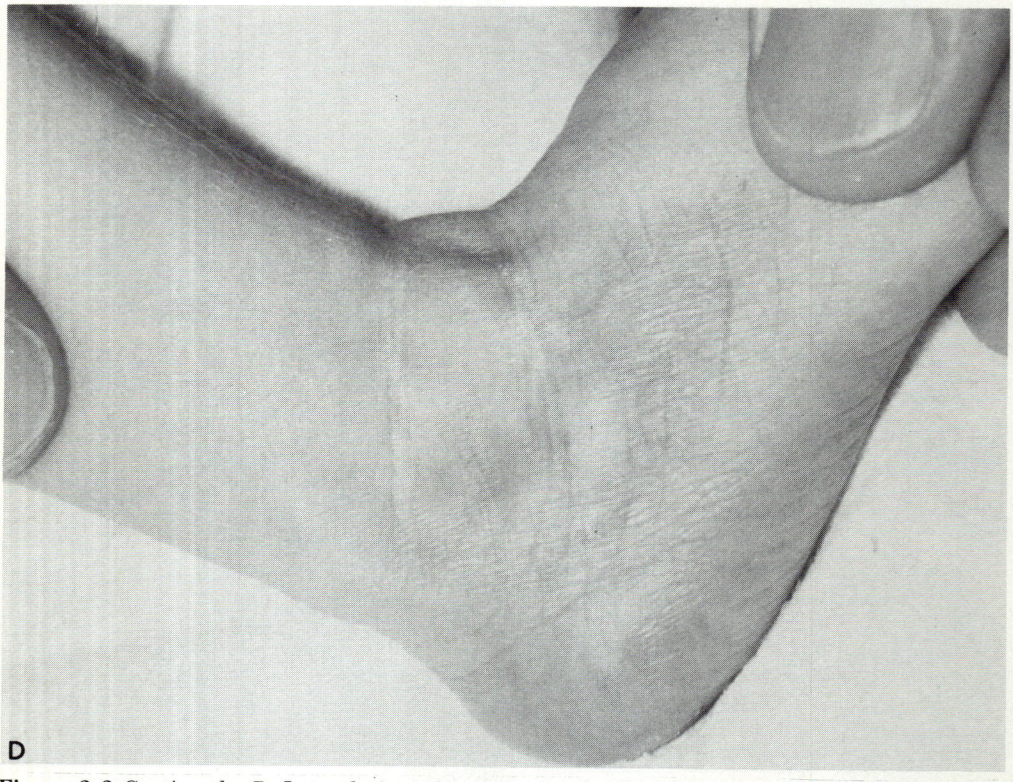

Figure 2–2 *Continued.* *D,* Lateral view of a ventriflexed calcaneovalgus foot showing the same type of features as in *C,* but less severe.

METATARSUS ADDUCTUS

1.2 METATARSUS ADDUCTUS

GENESIS. Compression of the forefoot with the legs flexed across the lower body in late gestation may be one cause of metatarsus adductus, which has a frequency of about 1.2 per thousand and an 80 per cent predilection for the male. This may be aggravated by the infant sleeping on the abdomen with the knees tucked up and the lower legs and feet rolled in.

FEATURES. The predominant feature is adduction of the forefoot, often with some supination. The ankle and heel are generally in normal position.

MANAGEMENT, PROGNOSIS, AND COUNSEL. For mild and flexible cases, manipulative stretch and avoidance of sleeping postures that tend to augment the deformity are all that are usually required. If, after several months, the sleeping posture is tending to augment the deformity, then attempts to change the posture may be of value. In the experience of Dr. Sig T. Hansen, Jr., at the University of Washington, several devices have been useful.[4] One is putting the child in a heavy sleeper, which keeps the child warm and causes him or her to sprawl rather than tuck in the legs. The leggings of the sleeper may be pinned or sewn together at the knees, making it difficult to achieve the deforming posture. If this is not helpful, a pair of open-toed straight-last shoes with the heels tied together may be placed on the child. If simpler measures fail, reversed-last open-toed shoes tied at the heels may be tried for night-time wear, or the shoes may be connected by a short Denis-Browne or Fillauer splint to provide mild outward rotation. It may be necessary to augment this by early reversed-last shoes in order to maintain the corrected form.

If, when first treated, the foot cannot be passively placed in the neutral position, it is generally wiser to achieve initial correction by very careful casting. If there is associated internal tibial torsion, as frequently happens, a long leg cast is utilized; however, if there is no internal tibial torsion, a short leg cast is usually adequate. The hindfoot and midfoot should be carefully maintained in their neutral positions during the casting. Early management may be critical, since the metatarsus adductus tends to become less flexible with time. The recurrence risk in first degree relatives is 1.8 per cent.[1]

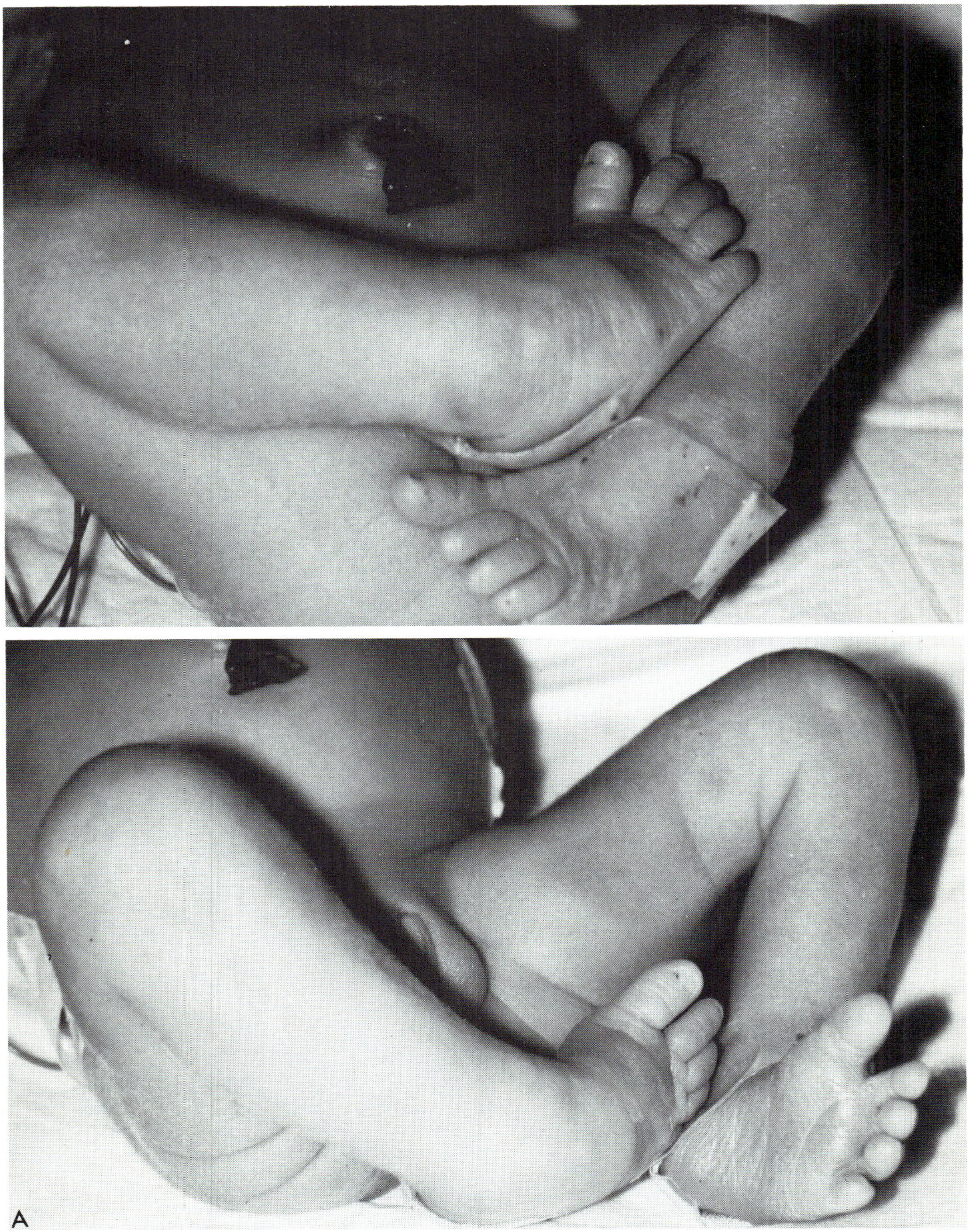

Figure 2–3. *A*, Presumed in-utero position (above), the "position of comfort," which engendered external constraint molding of right forefoot into the metatarsus adductus position shown below.

Illustration continued on following page

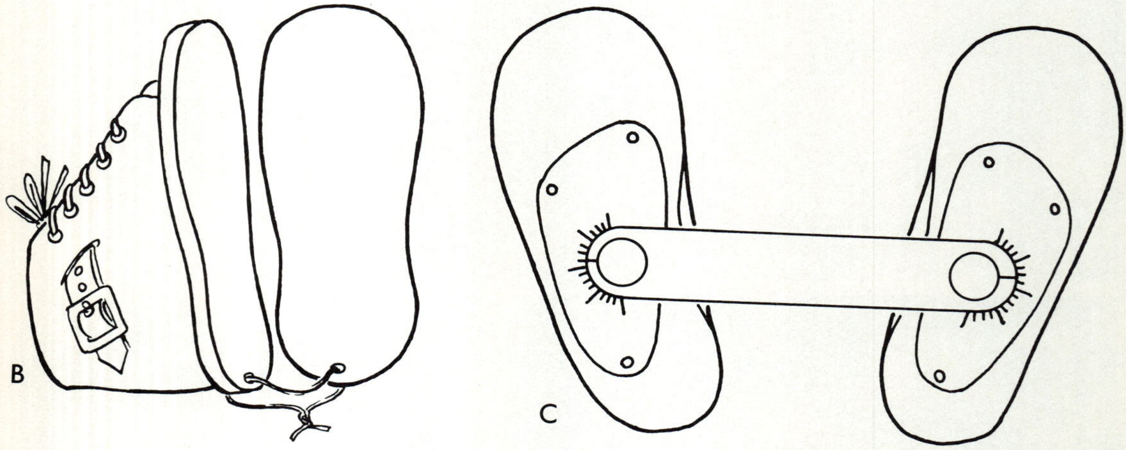

Figure 2–3 *Continued.* *B,* Simple method for controlling sleeping posture by using open-toed straight-last shoes and tying the heels together with a shoe lace through holes punched in the heels. *C,* Denis-Browne splint or similar Fillauer bar may be placed on sleeping shoes to prevent deforming sleeping posture. The bar should be relatively short.

EQUINOVARUS

1.3 EQUINOVARUS

("Clubfoot")

GENESIS. This is often a serious foot defect, with up to 50 per cent of cases requiring surgical intervention. Although it is not possible to state with assurance the proportion of equinovarus foot defects that represent constraint foot deformities, it is most likely about one third to one half of cases. The overall frequency is 1.2 per cent 1000,[1] but this varies among racial groups. For example, in Polynesians the frequency is 12 times higher.[2] The overall sex predilection is 2:1 in favor of the male. However, when the mild "postural equinovarus" cases are considered, there is about a 2:1 propensity toward the female.[1] The most common positional equinovarus deformity is considered to be the result of uterine constraint on the folded legs, especially in the situation of oligohydramnios.

FEATURES. The forefoot is inverted as are the heel and the whole foot, which is in plantar flexion. There is often a varus deformation of the neck of the talus and a medial shift of the navicular on the head of the talus. The calf muscles may be deficient with shortening. The fibrous capsules of the joints may be thickened on the lateral aspect of the foot. If there has been a long-term compression over the lateral margin of the foot, there may be a thin skin with a deficiency of subcutaneous tissue at that site.

MANAGEMENT, PROGNOSIS, AND COUNSEL. Early and rather rigorous management is merited. If there is some flexibility to the foot, initial manipulation and stretch taping toward dorsiflexion of the foot with eversion of the heel should be tried. Maintenance of the corrected position may sometimes need to be fostered by casting and/or Denis-Browne splints in order to prevent a lapse toward the deformed position. If continued improvement does not occur after one to three months of conservative management, or if there is little or no flexibility in the foot (especially the ability to bring the hindfoot equinus into a normal position), then early surgical intervention seems merited. About 40 to 50 per cent of cases arrive at surgery and about one third of this latter group are improved. If correction is not obtained by one year of age it is unlikely to be fully achieved. The surgery usually involves lengthening of the Achilles tendon, division of the posterior ankle capsule talofibular ligament, and release of the tibialis posterior, flexor hallucis, and digitorum longus if they are unduly tight.

There has not been a clear separation of postural equinovarus and non-constraint–induced equinovarus. From my experience, I believe the prognosis for restoration toward normal form is much better when the cause is uterine constraint in an otherwise normal child. The general recurrence risk for equinovarus defect is 3 per cent.[1] When only the postural equinovarus cases are considered, the recurrence risk is 2.6 per cent.[1]

DIFFERENTIAL DIAGNOSIS. The etiology for the type that is not constraint induced, has a predilection for males, and varies in racial incidence is unknown. It tends to be more rigid than constraint induced deformation, and there is more likely to be atrophy of calf muscles. The talus tends to be hypoplastic and altered in form. There is even a question whether the primary defect may not be in the talonavicular development.

When equinovarus is a feature of neuromuscular disorders, limb deficiency, or a skeletal dysplasia, the prognosis for achieving a normal form to the foot is usually poor. Equinovarus foot position is a not uncommon accompaniment of certain neurological deficiencies, especially the spinal cord defect that occurs so frequently with meningomyelocele. An infant with equinovarus defect not only should be checked for the obvious meningomyelocele but should also be given a close inspection of the lower spine for hemangiomata, hairy nevus, or other subtle clues to an underlying spinal cord defect. A cautious neurological evaluation is also indicated. Partial degrees of equinovarus position occur in a number of cerebral palsy disorders. Deficiency of the tibia (tibial hemimelia) often results in an equinovarus foot defect. One or more amniotic bands around the leg, proximal to the foot, may result in an equinovarus foot. The defect may be part of an arthrogryposis disorder such as amyoplasia, in which the inward rotation of the hands and shoulders may allow for an overall diagnosis. Finally, equinovarus may be one feature of a skeletal dysplasia such as diastrophic dwarfism, a syndrome that includes small stature with short limbs, unduly short thumbs, and hypertrophy of ear cartilage.

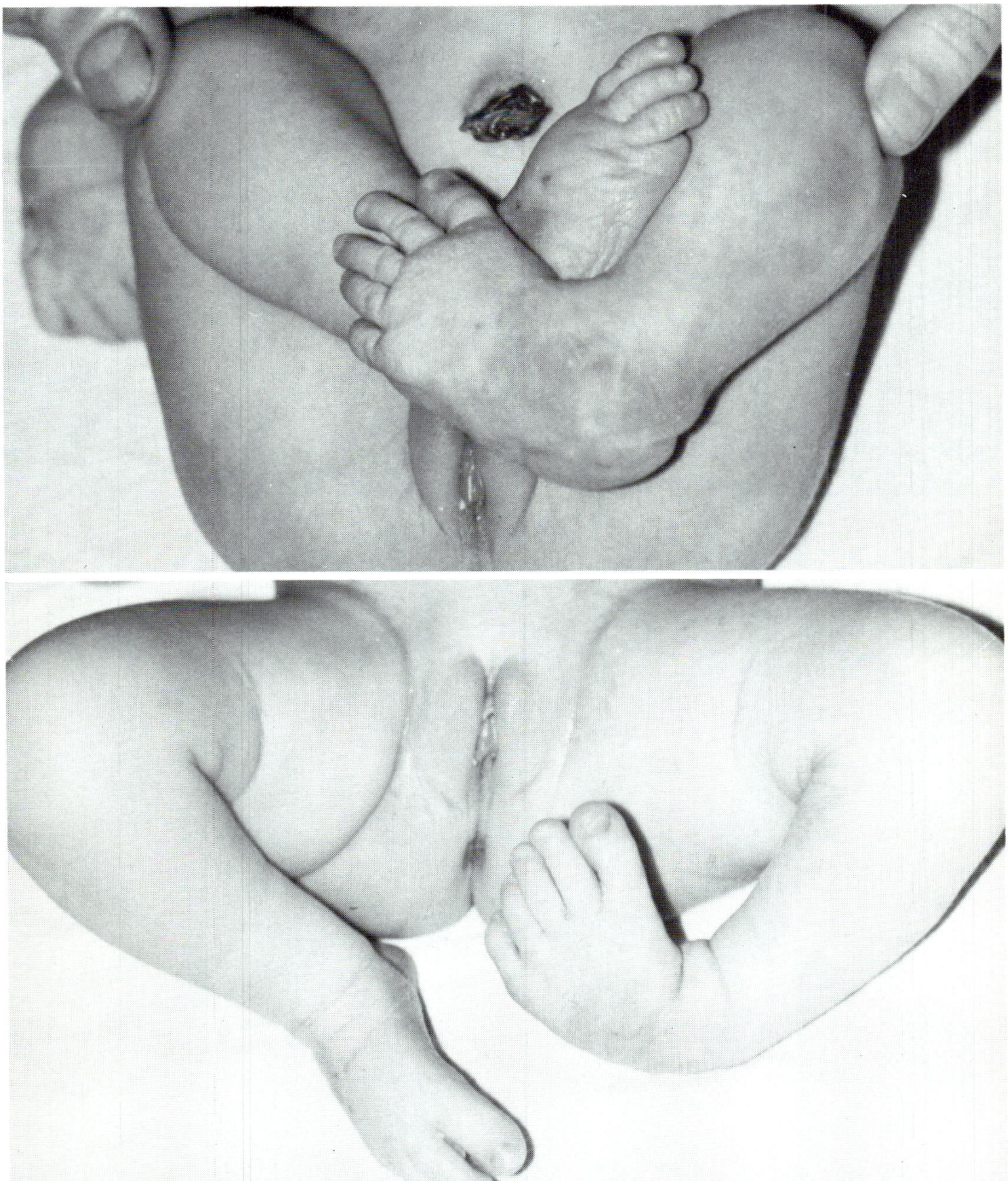

Figure 2–4. Equinovarus. *A,* Presumed in-utero position that engendered the equinovarus deformation of the left foot. At the site of in-utero compression over the left lateral ankle the skin is very thin with a fine erythematous reaction, secondary to prolonged pressure.

Illustration continued on following page

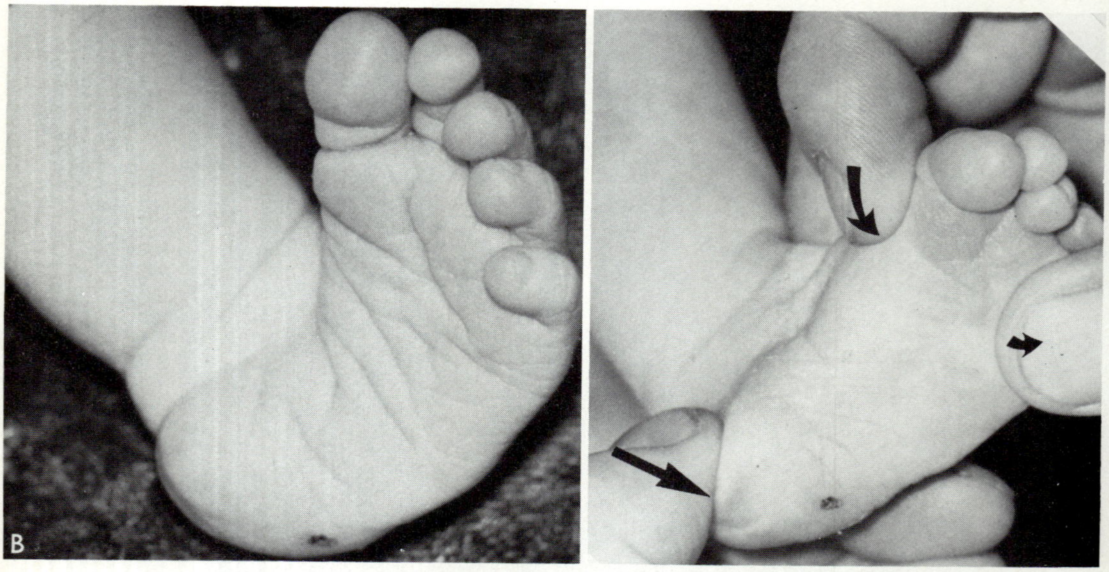

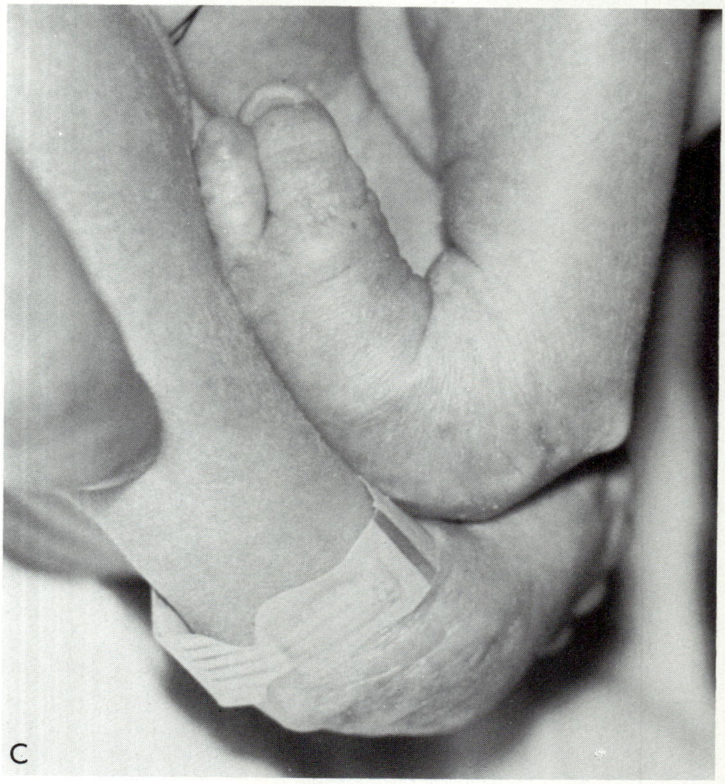

Figure 2–4 *Continued.* *B,* Plantar view of an equinovarus foot. Note the inward rotation of the heel and forefoot with the whole foot deviated inward at the ankle. Outward pressure on the heel and forefoot resulted in partial correction toward a neutral foot positioning. These feet were corrected by taping and manipulation alone. *C,* Presumed in-utero position that yielded rather severe equinovarus deformation by birth. Note the prominent lateral malleolus over which the skin was very thin, implying pressure constraint.

Illustration continued on opposite page

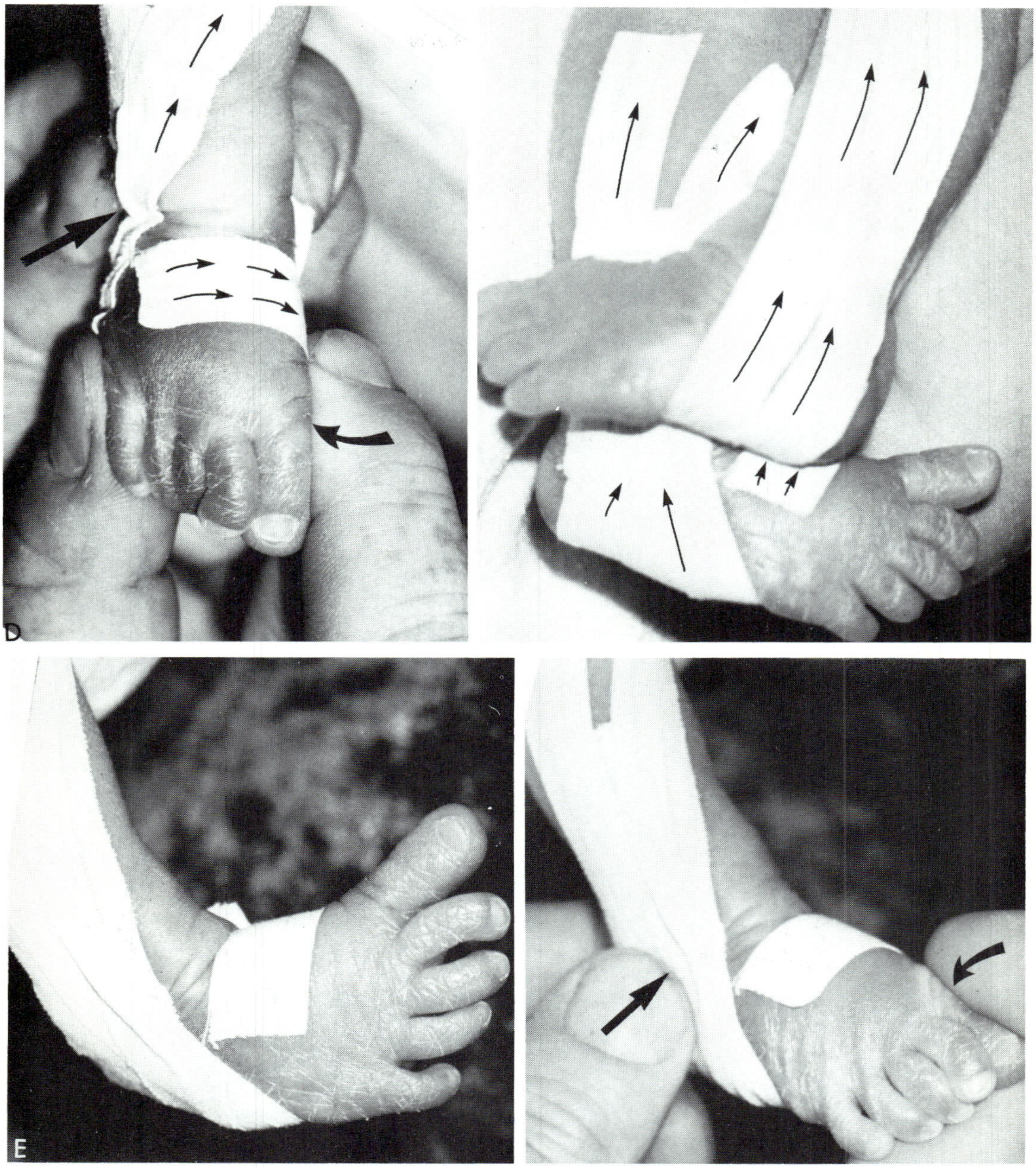

Figure 2–4 *Continued.* *D,* After manipulating the foot of the patient shown in *C* into a more normal position, several layers of adhesive tape are applied (tincture of benzoin on skin), starting over the dorsum of the foot and bringing the tape medialward under the sole and up the lateral side of the leg. After taping, the feet tend to return partially to their pretaped position, as shown to the right. *E,* When the foot is taped and partially corrected, it is possible for the parents to repeatedly manipulate the foot toward the ideal position, a mode of management that is not possible when the foot is in a cast.

1.4 DEFORMED TOES

GENESIS. Constraint of the feet while the legs are in a flexed and folded position can result in the medial overlapping of the toes, especially the fifth, fourth, and third.

FEATURES. The fifth, fourth, and third toes tend to overlap medially with mild to moderate incurvature. There may be accentuated longitudinal creasing in the sole of the foot where it has been "folded" by external compression.

MANAGEMENT AND PROGNOSIS. If the toes do not readily tend to realign after birth, then manipulative lateral stretching and/or taping is merited. Rarely is later surgery necessary.

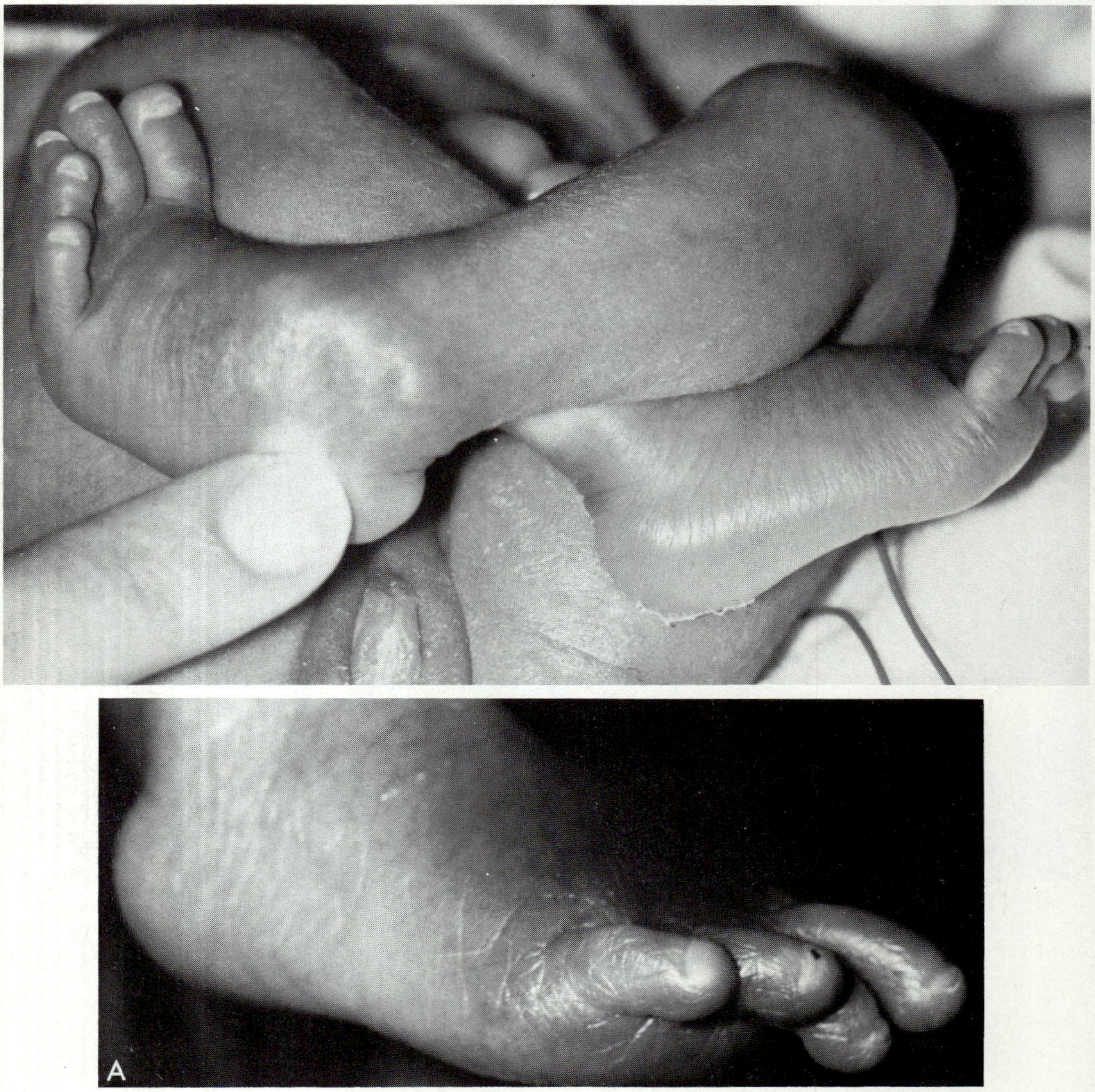

Figure 2–5. Deformed toes. *A*, Presumed position in utero in which uterine constraint compressed the forefeet resulting in overlapping of the toes.

Illustration continued on oppoiste page

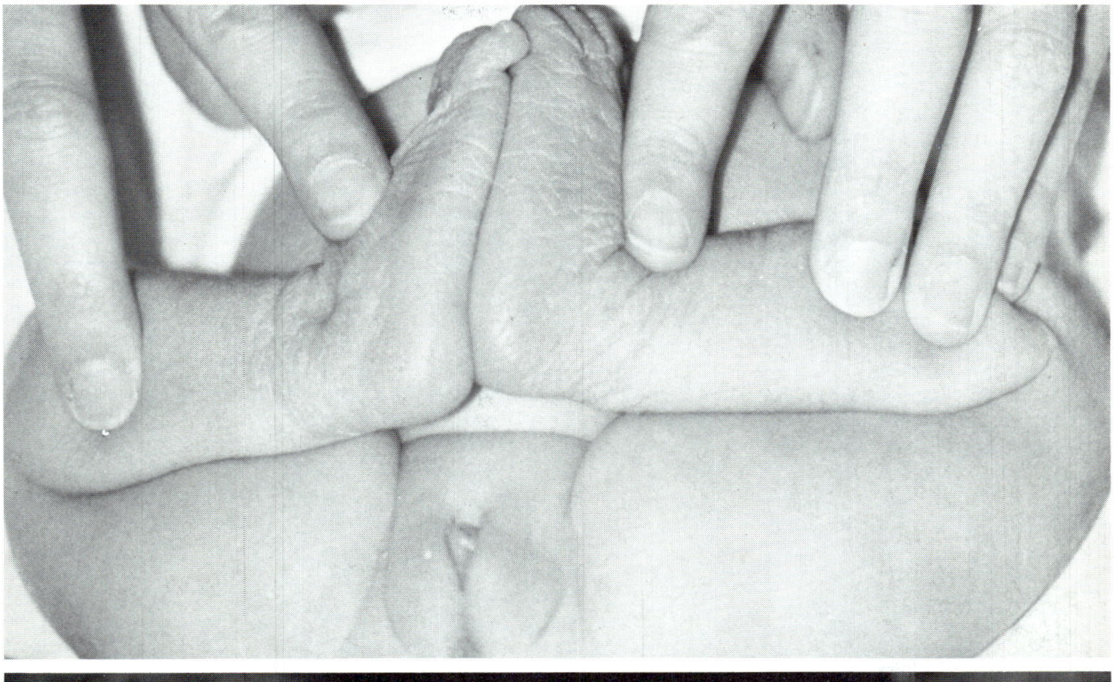

Figure 2–5 *Continued.* *B,* Presumed positioning in utero in which uterine constraint compressed the feet, yielding unilateral partially folded forefoot and deformation of toes. Note the thin, wrinkled skin over the lateral malleolus (to viewer's left), which is a strong clue that constraint induction of the deformation occurred.

2. TIBIAL TORSION

(Tibial Inbowing)

GENESIS. Torsion of the tibia is sufficiently common in the normal newborn to be considered a normal variant. However, unusual degrees of this inbowing occur in about 3 per cent of newborns and is especially likely with constraint of the legs in the folded and flexed position. For this apparent reason it is a frequent feature in positional equinovarus deformity, which derives from similar mechanical constraint.

FEATURES. The tibia is medially rotated, with the most acute incurving being distally. This tends to angle the plantar surfaces of the feet toward each other. There may also be mild to moderate pes varus in association with medial tibial "torsion."

MANAGEMENT, PROGNOSIS, AND COUNSEL. Seldom is any management required. Following release from the constraint there tends to be progressive straightening of the legs. However, sleeping posture may tend to foster persistence of the tibial torsion. The same preventive measures for sleeping posture as mentioned for metatarsus adductus may be employed. If tibial torsion persists into the second year, night splinting may be indicated.

DIFFERENTIAL DIAGNOSIS. The lower legs may be more bowed than usual because of a neuromuscular disorder such as meningomyelocele. Problems in bone formation may also result in malleable or fragile bones, such as occur with hypophosphatasia (malleable) and osteogenesis imperfecta (fragile).

3.0 JOINT DISLOCATION, ESPECIALLY OF HIP

GENERAL. Joints normally develop secondarily within the condensed mesenchyme that will form the bones. Hence a dislocated joint always represents a displacement of the bone from the original site of the joint. Once a joint has been dislocated it is obvious that the joint capsule has been stretched into unusual form and that any ligamentous attachment, such as the ligamentum teres of the hip joint, has been elongated and deformed. If the dislocation is of sufficient duration, the aberrant forces will alter the form of the original joint socket. The occurrence of dislocation is dependent on at least three factors, as shown in Figure 2–6. The joint that is most liable to dislocation is the hip joint because of the major forces that may be brought to bear on it by such situations as breech position in later fetal life and because of the sloping angulation of the acetabulum. The second most common dislocation is of the proximal head of the radius, and the third most common dislocation is at the knee, yielding a genu recurvatum. Because of the relative importance and frequency of dislocation of the hip, it will be given more extensive coverage.

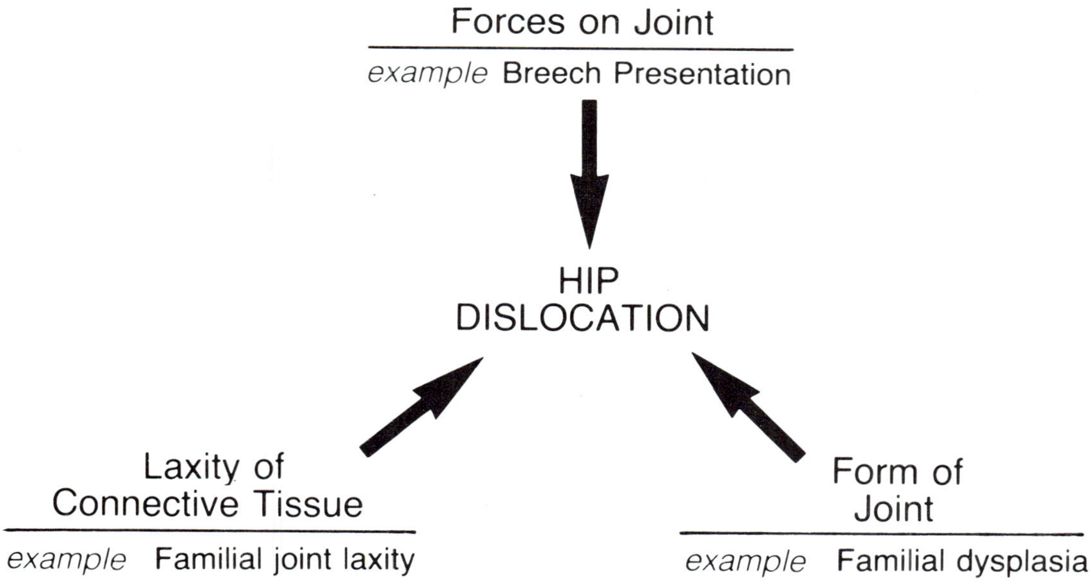

Figure 2–6. Factors that interact in the genesis of joint dislocation, with examples that relate to hip dislocation.

3.1 HIP DISLOCATION

GENESIS. Figure 2–6 depicts some of the interacting factors that relate to the genesis of hip dislocation. Laxity of connective tissue is an important factor. The 4:1 to 5:1 predilection toward the female is considered to be the consequence of the female fetus being more lax than the male fetus.

Arena and Smith[1] suggested that this is the consequence of a lack of testosterone effect in the female fetus. Testosterone, present in the male fetus, results in tougher connective tissue. This has been demonstrated in the hip capsule of the young rodent.[2] Dunn[3] has shown the excess of dislocation of the hip in the female to be as high as 13:1 when it is an isolated deformation. However, when there are multiple deformations, the sex ratio is closer to equality. A heritable tendency toward increased joint laxity is another factor that has been recognized. Carter and Wilkinson[4] found that laxity of three or more joints, noted in 7 per cent of individuals overall, was present in 22 per cent of the first-degree relatives of sporadic cases of dislocation of the hip. When there were multiple cases of dislocation of the hip in a family, an impressive 65 per cent of first degree relatives had undue joint laxity.[4]

The forces that tend to thrust the head of the femur out of the acetabulum cause a stretching of the joint capsule and of the ligamentum teres. These forces are most commonly the result of constraint in late fetal life. Since these forces are more likely to affect the first offspring, dislocation of the hip is more common in the first born. Certain positions in the crowded environment during late gestation are particularly likely to cause dislocation of the hip. Breech position is notorious in this respect. About 50 per cent of cases of hip dislocation had been in the breech position in utero.[3] In all breech term births (about 3.5 per cent of births) there is a 17 per cent frequency of dislocation of the hip, and for breech with extended legs in utero (frank breech) the incidence is 25 per cent.[3] The breech position with the buttocks in the maternal pelvis and the fetal hips tightly flexed upon the abdomen tends to mechanically cause a lever thrust of the femoral head out of the acetabulum, especially when the legs are extended and "caught" between the abdomen of the fetus and the uterine wall.

The fact that the fetus more commonly lies with its left side toward the mother's spine may be responsible for the increased propensity of the left hip to be dislocated rather than the right.[3]

Oligohydramnios, causing overall constraint of the fetus, is associated with an increased frequency of hip dislocation, at least partially the consequence of the increased frequency of breech position with oligohydramnios.

The position of the infant *after birth* is also important in the genesis of dislocation of the hip. The hip joint may be lax at birth and only become dislocated postnatally.[5] Undue leg extension in early infancy is considered a factor in the postnatal genesis of hip dislocation.[4] Thus, the hip that has been flexed with a relatively contracted psoas muscle in utero is more likely to be thrust out of its socket by forced extension of the leg. The increased frequency of dislocation of the hip in American Indians and in the Lapps has been at least partially attributed to their practice of swaddling young infants with the legs extended. On the other hand, the relatively low incidence of hip dislocation in the Hong Kong Chinese has been attributed to the mothers' custom of carrying the babies on their lower back with the hips flexed and partially abducted, which mechanically favors maintenance of the femoral head in the acetabulum.

All gradations of dislocation from partially stretched dislocatable hip to fully dislocated hip occur with an overall frequency of about 1 per cent. Considering the full spectrum, Barlow[6] observed that 60 per cent of these dislocatable hips are stable in the normal location by one week of age and 88 per cent are stable by two months of age. The remaining 12 per cent represents frank dislocation of the hip that was evident at birth or during early infancy, a frequency of 1.2 per 1000.

FEATURES. The usual direction of the dislocation is posterior. The major problem with dislocation of the hip is that it is seldom readily evident on gross inspection of the newly born baby and may not *become* evident until early postnatal life. Thus, delineation of the features involves a cautious physical examination, searching for signs of the whole dislocation spectrum, from a lax dislocatable hip to the dislocated hip that can still be relocated into the acetabulum to the dislocated hip that cannot be relocated. The following type of hip examination is warranted for all newborn babies.

It is of utmost importance that the infant be relaxed during the hip examination. A pacifier or bottle may be of value in this regard. With the infant in the supine position and the hips and knees flexed to 90 degrees and mildly abducted, the examiner, who is facing the baby's buttocks, grasps each thigh. The thumb of each hand is placed on the medial part of the upper thigh and the third finger is placed over the lateral aspect of the upper thigh at the level of the greater trochanter. The first maneuver is to pull out quite gently on the thigh and at the same time push the upper thigh medialward with the third finger. If the hip is dislocated posteriorly — the usual direction for dislocation — and can be relocated, the examiner will feel a noticeable "clunk" as the femoral head slips over the acetabular shelf and into the acetabular socket. If the result of this maneuver is negative, then the second maneuver is to pull out gently on the thigh while at the same time pushing the upper thigh lateralward with the thumb. If this results in a noticeable (palpable) "clunk," as the femoral head is forced over the acetabular rim into a posteriorly dislocated position, the hip may be referred to as dislocatable. (It may also be referred to as an unstable hip.) Minor clicks may be noted in about one third of the examinations and do not appear to be of any consequence. Rather, it is the palpable "clunk" or "thunk" that is relevant.

It is *most* important to appreciate that neither of these above maneuvers will be positive for the hip that is dislocated and cannot be manually relocated. This hip will usually show a limitation in abduction; the greater trochanter may be felt to be posteriorly and superiorly displaced; and the upper leg may appear relatively short. When the dislocation is unilateral or asymmetrical in degree, there may be asymmetry in the relative length of the legs, though the lower legs and feet are the same length. There may also be an obvious discrepancy in the creases of the thigh folds between the two sides. The same type of examination is indicated in the first one or two postnatal examinations after discharge from the newborn nursery. At this time the prior maneuvers, which are routine in the newborn, are of relatively little value. It is paramount to appreciate that not all dislocation of the hip is detected in the newborn nursery and that detectional surveillance during early infancy is merited.[5] Roentgenograms, which are of little value in the newborn because of the incomplete ossification of the acetabulum and lack of ossification in the femoral head, become more valuable after several months of age in order to detect evidence of dislocation when clinical suspicion of such a problem exists.

A number of aberrations in morphogenesis may occur as secondary features to dislocation of the hip. They are dependent on the age of development and the duration and extent of the dislocation. These include deformation of the femoral head, imperfect articular cartilage, adherence between the articular surface of the femoral head and the capsular tissue, short psoas, adductor, and hamstring muscles, anteversion at the hip, development of a false acetabulum, and elongated ligamentum teres and stretched joint capsule. When such changes are profound, it may be difficult or even impossible to accomplish a closed replacement of the femoral head into its original acetabulum.

MANAGEMENT, PROGNOSIS, AND COUNSEL. Early and simple conservative management of dislocation of the hip will usually result in a normal hip by the age of walking. If dislocation of the hip is discovered after one year of age, the condition usually requires prolonged and complicated management and results in varying degrees of lifelong disability. Hence early diagnosis, emphasized above, is a key to successful management.

The most common hip diagnosis at birth is the dislocatable or unstable hip. Even though the femoral head is in a normal position at birth, it is considered best to provide prophylactic splinting of the dislocatable hip in order to prevent the very real possibility of insidious hip dislocation in early infancy. Such splinting is continued until the hip becomes firmly held in place by its own connective tissue, which had been stretched prior to birth. The aim of the splinting is to maintain the femoral head in the acetabulum with reliable but not excessive constraint The recommended position is with the hips flexed about 90 degrees and abducted about 25 to 30 degrees. The full frogleg position has been discouraged because the constant rather excessive forcing of the femoral head into the acetabulum may occasionally result in avascular necrosis in the head of the immobilized femur. There have been a variety of types of splints employed. Probably a pillow splint is not reliable enough. A soft, easily cleaned splint, such as the Plastizote splint, is usually preferable. For the dislocatable hip a period of four to six weeks of splinting is usually adequate to yield a "tight" hip.

The dislocated hip that can be relocated should be splinted in the above manner, with assurance that the femoral head is staying in the acetabulum. For this hip, the Pavlik splint may be preferable. The duration of splinting varies with the severity of the problem and the age at diagnosis. When detected at birth to one month of age, the mean duration of splinting is 3.6 months, and at one to three months it is seven months. If the dislocation was not detected until three to six months, the mean duration of splinting is 9.3 months.

If it is not possible to manually reduce the dislocation, leg traction should be utilized in an effort to lengthen the contracted muscles and hopefully allow for a closed reduction. If this is not possible, surgical correction is merited. Surgery may include the lengthening or detachment of contracted muscles and reconstruction of the distorted joint capsule. Surgery is often postponed until the infant is about a year old because of the risk of ischemic necrosis following earlier hip surgery.

Uncorrected dislocation of the hip will adversely affect walking. There is usually a pronounced waddling limp and the later development of degenerative hip problems with chronic disability.

The recurrence risk for the more common type of dislocation of the hip is in the range of 3 to 6 per cent, being higher when a boy is affected than when a girl is affected.[4] If both a parent and a child are affected the recurrence risk may be as high as 30 per cent.

DIFFERENTIAL DIAGNOSIS. A malformation problem that itself enhances the likelihood of breech position, or a malformation problem that leads to oligohydramnios (and thereby both excess constraint and enhanced breech positioning), is associated with an increased frequency of dislocation of the hip secondary to the more primary malformation problem.

A number of neurological disorders may lead to dislocation of the hip, presumably on the basis of diminished muscle strength in holding the femoral head into the acetabulum and/or muscular imbalance. Thus dislocation of the hip may be secondary to meningomyelocele and may occur in certain categories of cerebral palsy, especially when there is flexion and/or adduction spasm at the hip.

In certain types of arthrogryposis (multiple joint contractures) there may be dislocation of the hip. One specific clinical entity in which it occurs is amyoplasia congenita.

Finally, there are a number of syndromes in which dislocation of the hip occurs as a frequent or occasional defect. One of the most striking of these is the Larsen syndrome, in which there tend to be multiple joint dislocations plus an unusually low nasal bridge.

REFERENCES

General

Lloyd Roberts, G.C.: Orthopaedics in infancy and childhood. New York, Appleton-Century-Crofts, 1971, p. 337.

Staheli, L.T.: Congenital dislocation of the hip. Perinatal Care *2*:14, 1978.

Specific

1. Arena, F., and Smith, D. W.: Sex liability to single structural defects. Am. J. Dis. Child. *132*:970, 1978.
2. Hama, H., Yamamuro, T., and Takeda, T.: Experimental studies on connective tissue of the capsular ligament. Acta Orthop. Scand. *47*:473, 1976.
3. Dunn, P.M: Perinatal observations on the etiology of congenital dislocation of the hip. Clin. Orthop. *119*:11, 1976.
4. Carter, C.O., and Wilkinson, J.A.: Genetic and environmental factors in the etiology of congenital dislocation of the hip. Clin. Orthop. Rel. Res. *33*:March-April, 1964.
5. Place, M., Parkin, P.M., and Fitton, M.: Effectiveness of neonatal screening for congenital dislocation of the hip. Lancet *2*:249, 1978.
6. Barlow, T.G.: Early diagnosis and treatment of congenital dislocation of the hip. J. Bone Joint Surg. *44B*:292, 1962.
7. Hensinger, R.N.: Congenital dislocation of the hip. Clin. Symposia *31*:3, 1979.

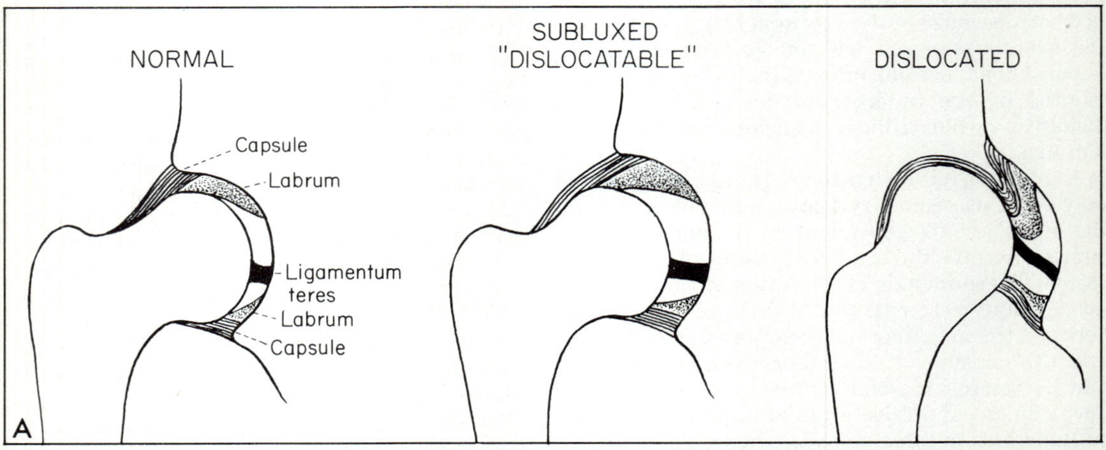

Figure 2–7. *A*, The normal hip, the moderately stretched "dislocatable" hip, and the overly stretched dislocated hip. (From Clarren, S., and Smith, D. W.: Congenital deformities. Pediatr. Clin. North Amer. *24*:665, 1977.)

Illustration continued on opposite page

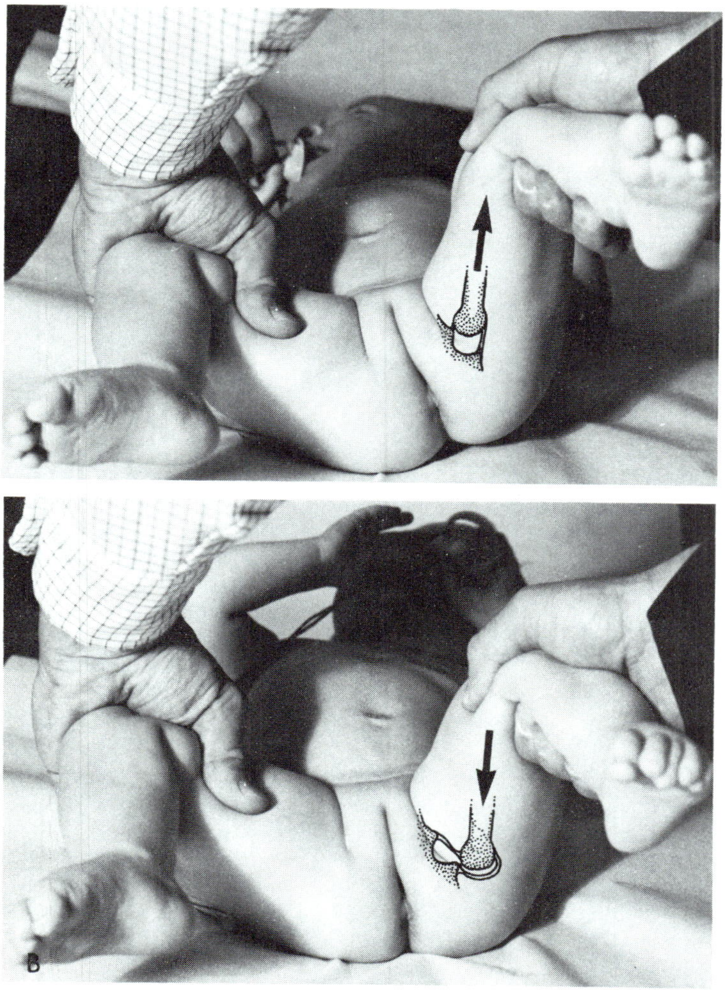

Figure 2-7 *Continued.* *B,* Technique of Barlow maneuver, which assists in detecting the unstable dislocatable hip, which is in the acetabulum. The leg is forcibly pulled up during the upper maneuver. Passage over the rim usually yields a noticeable "clunk." (Courtesy of Dr. Lynn Staheli, University of Washington.)

Illustration continued on following page

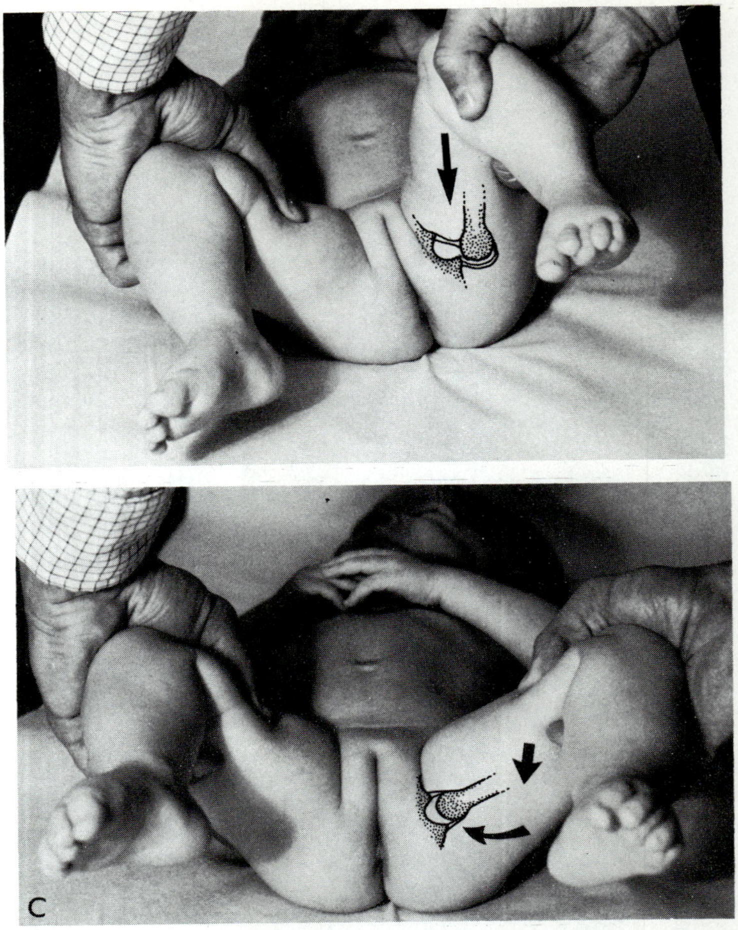

C

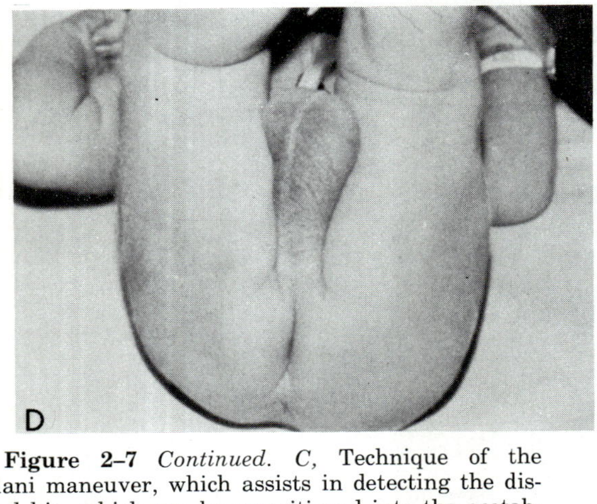

D

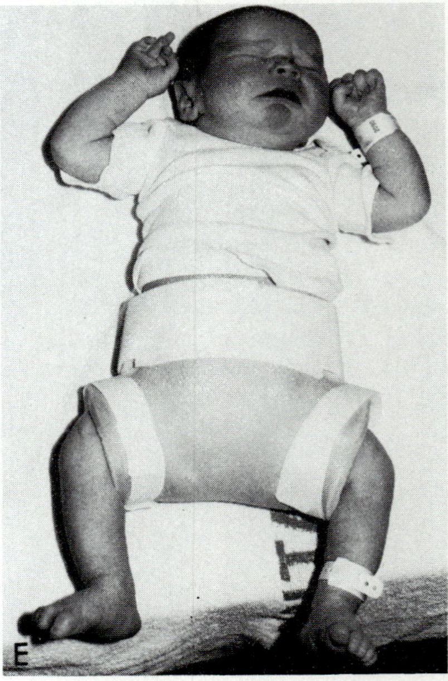

E

Figure 2–7 *Continued. C,* Technique of the Ortolani maneuver, which assists in detecting the dislocated hip, which can be repositioned into the acetabulum. Above, downward pressure further dislocates the hip; below, inward rotation of the hip will force the femoral head over the acetabular rim, leading to a noticeable "clunk." *D,* Dislocated right hip in a young infant, evident by gross inspection. (Courtesy of Dr. Marylin Higginbottom, University of California at San Diego.) *E,* Plastizote splint utilized for the dislocatable hip in early infancy.

Illustration continued on opposite page

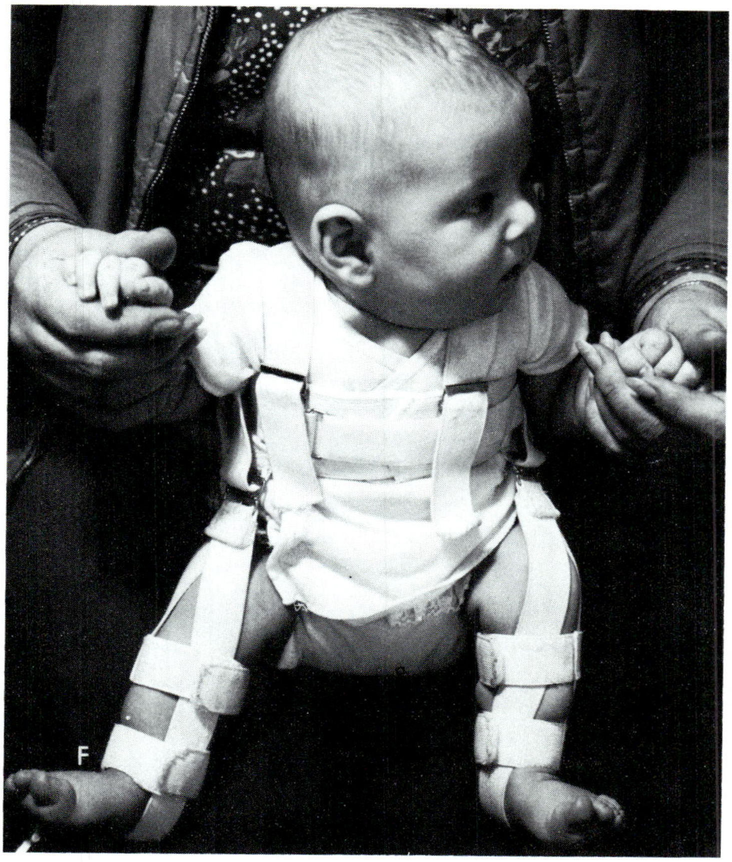

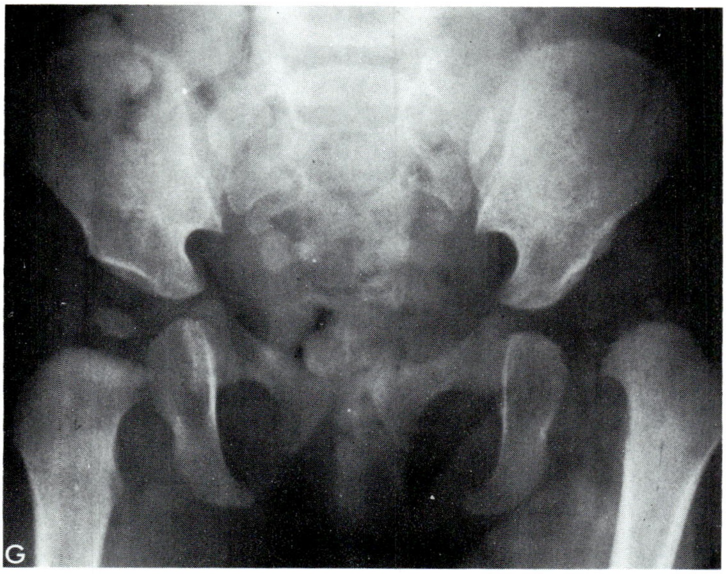

Figure 2–7 *Continued. F,* Pavlik splint used for maintaining reposition of the dislocated hip in early infancy. *G,* The secondary changes in acetabulum and neck of femur plus the unseen hour-glass elongation of the hip capsule, elongated ligamentum teres, and foreshortened muscle attachments relating to long-term dislocation of the hip. (Figures *B, C, D, E,* and *F* are courtesy of Dr. Lynn Staheli, Head of Pediatric Orthopedics, Children's Orthopedic Hospital, Seattle.)

3.2 KNEE DISLOCATION

(Genu Recurvatum)

GENESIS. Hyperextension of the leg with dislocation at the knee most commonly derives from the legs being in extended posture in the breech position. Unusual constraint in a bicornuate uterus and other modes may produce it as well.

FEATURES. "Backward" curvature of the knee with an unstable and sometimes dislocated knee. The quadriceps muscle tends to be short, and the distal quadriceps may be relatively fibrotic. The patella, a sesamoid bone which normally forms in the quadriceps tendon in response to stress, may be small or absent because of the lack of tension on the quadriceps tendon.

MANAGEMENT, PROGNOSIS, AND COUNSEL. Early adhesive strapping or casting in a corrected position may suffice to bring about a correction by eight weeks or so in about half of the cases. Recalcitrant cases usually require quadriceps lengthening and sometimes surgical correction of the stretched knee joint capsule and its attachments.

DIFFERENTIAL DIAGNOSIS. Similar to that for dislocation of the hip, but knee dislocation is less likely to occur with neurological disorders.

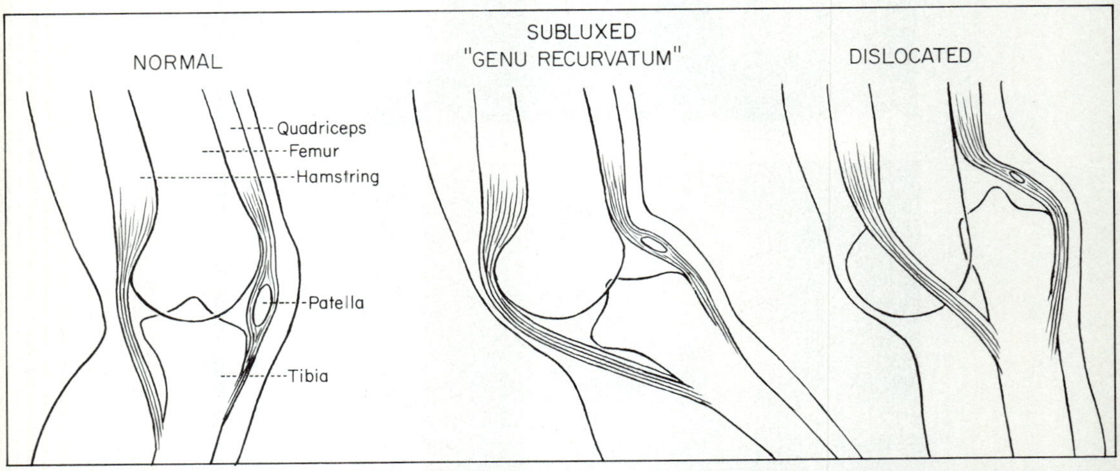

Figure 2–8. Normal knee, stretched tissues to the point of a subluxed "genu recurvatum" (most commonly occurring in prolonged frank breech position) and dislocated knee. The patella develops as a sesamoid bone in the tendon of the quadriceps muscle. With less tension, the sesamoid bone may be small to absent. (From Clarren, S. K., and Smith, D. W.: Congenital deformities. Pediat. Clin. North Amer. *24*:665, 1977.)

3.3 DISLOCATION OF THE RADIAL HEAD

GENERAL. The posterior and lateralward dislocation of the proximal head of the radius resulting in inability to fully supinate at the elbow generally gives rise to little disability and is seldom treated. Its genesis is seldom appreciated, although it most commonly occurs in association with dislocation of the hip.

NEUROPRAXIAS

4. NEUROPRAXIAS

(Palsies)

GENESIS. Prolonged compression of a peripheral nerve may lead to palsy, sometimes apparently on the basis of neural ischemia. The frequency of occurrence is about 1.4 per 1000.

FEATURES

Face. Facial nerve palsy secondary to compression of facial nerve. Also, ptosis of the eyelid has been observed.

Arm. Radial nerve compression between the humerus and rib cage when there is tight crowding in late gestation may lead to wrist drop (Erb's palsy).

Leg. Sciatic compression may cause weakness in one or both legs.

MANAGEMENT AND PROGNOSIS. There is usually little need for management. When the nerve compression has occurred in late gestation there is usually a full return of function within a matter of days to weeks. If the nerve compression occurs in early fetal life the consequences are more likely to be permanent, as delineated in disorder number 20.

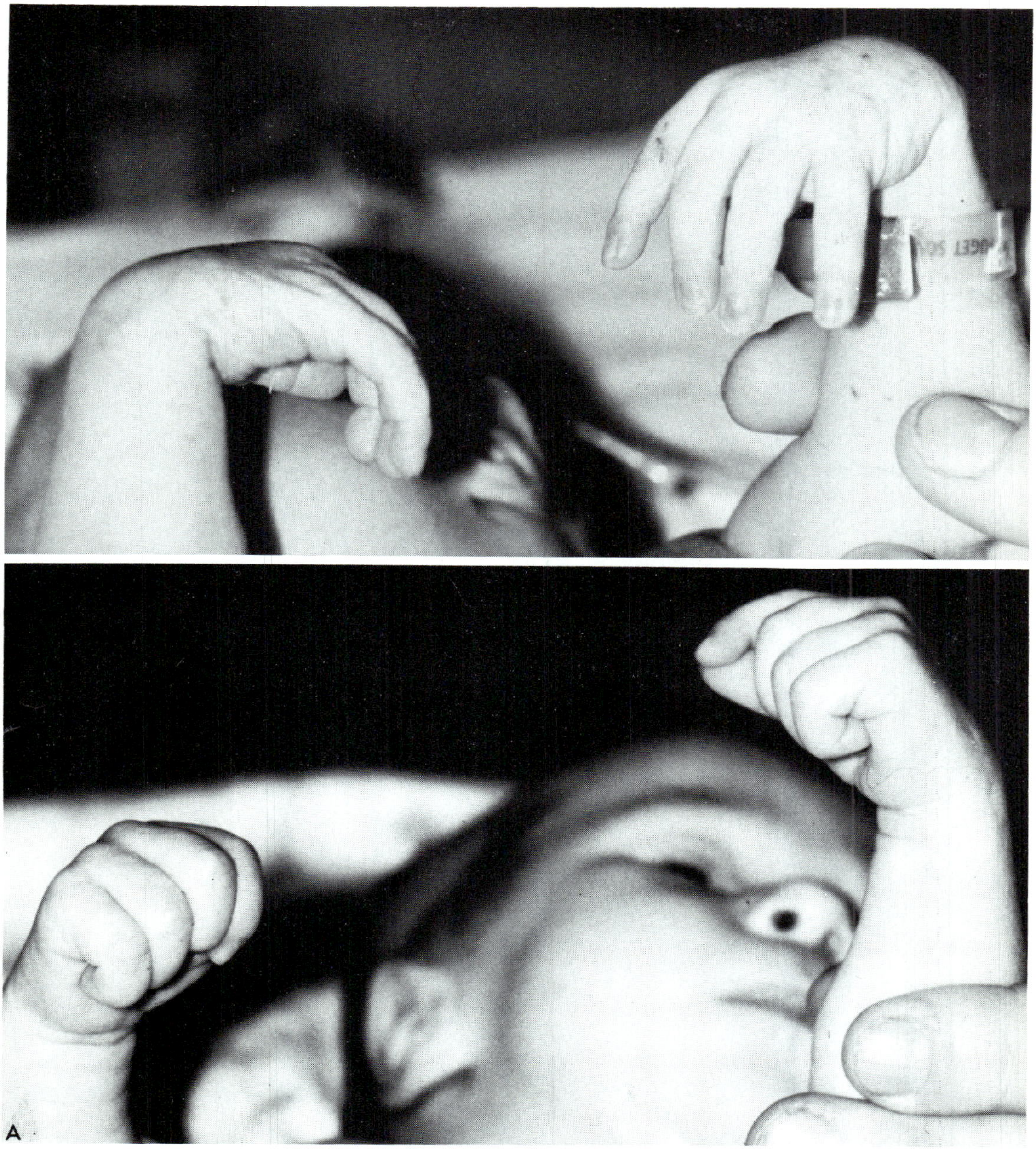

Figure 2–9. *A*, Top, Maximum extension of hands at birth. Erb's palsy secondary to constraint of radial nerve between the humerus and the rib cage. Bottom, Same infant at two months of age showing vast improvement in ability to extend the hand at the wrist and to clench the hand.

Illustration continued on following page

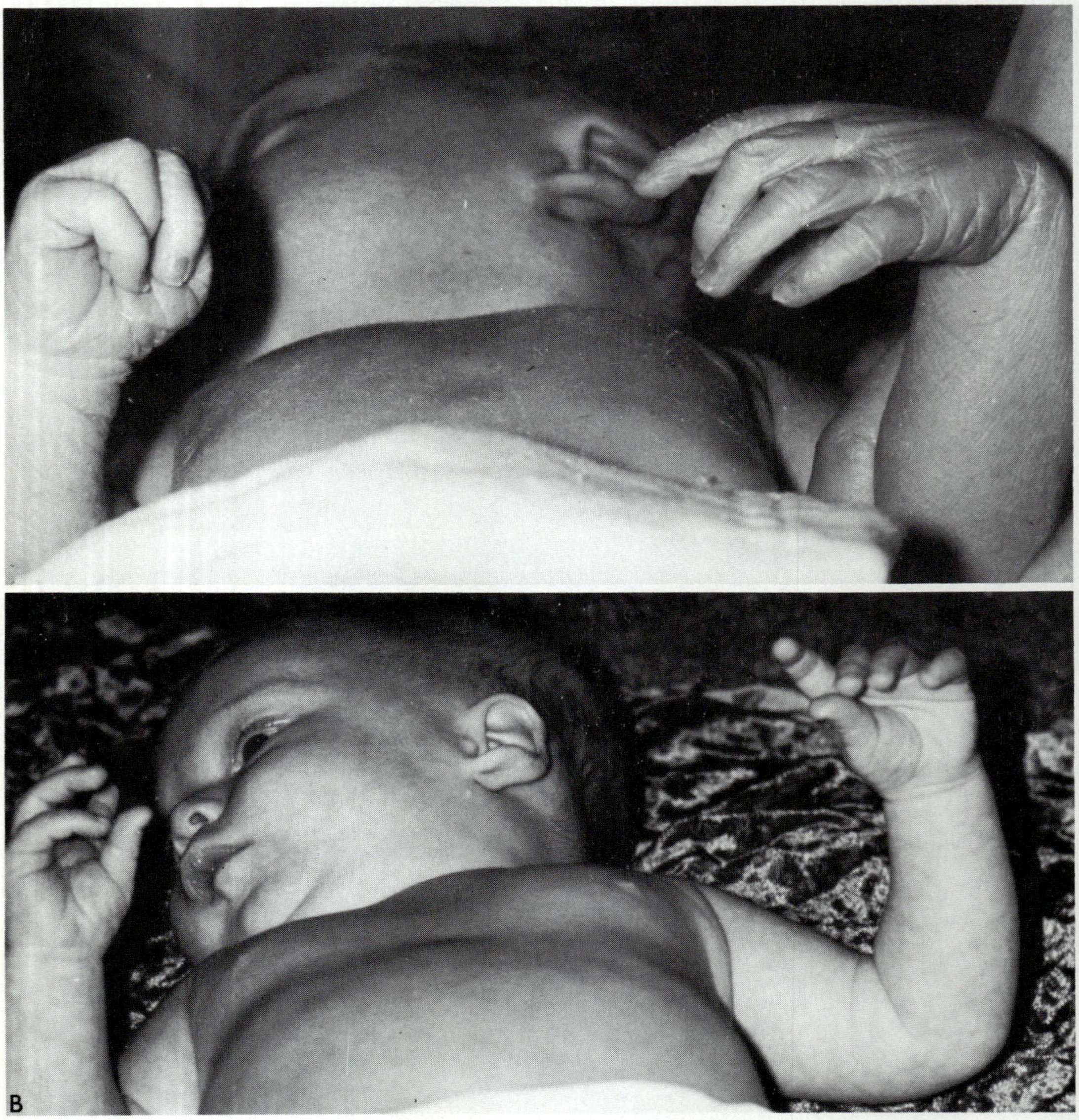

Figure 2–9 *Continued.* *B,* Unilateral Erb's palsy relating to compression at birth (above) and 12 weeks later, by which time function was normal. The compression in this instance related to engagement five weeks prior to delivery in a restricted birth canal.

5. THORACIC CAGE AND SPINE

5.1 LUNG HYPOPLASIA

GENESIS. Constraint of thoracic cage expansion by such causes as oligohydramnios or small uterine cavity.

FEATURES. Pulmonary hypoplasia with limited alveolar development. Liable to respiratory insufficiency with hyaline membrane development.

MANAGEMENT AND PROGNOSIS. When the thoracic compression has been the result of chronic leakage of amniotic fluid or a small uterine cavity, every measure toward oxygenation should be taken in the hope of maintaining survival until lung development becomes adequate for normal respiration.

DIFFERENTIAL DIAGNOSIS. Oligohydramnios may be the result of inadequate urine flow into the amniotic space, in which case the prognosis is usually grim.

Diaphragmatic hernia not only limits lung development on the side of the hernia but also shifts the mediastinal contents toward the opposite side and thereby limits lung growth on that side as well. Hence infants with this condition usually expire of respiratory insufficiency due to lung hypoplasia.

There are several skeletal dysplasias in which there is a profound impact on thoracic cage growth and thereby respiratory insufficiency. One is thanatophoric dwarfism. The word thanatophoric means "death dealing," and the death in this condition is usually the consequence of respiratory insufficiency. Even with achondroplasia there may be enough of a problem in thoracic growth to give rise to mild to moderate respiratory insufficiency at birth.

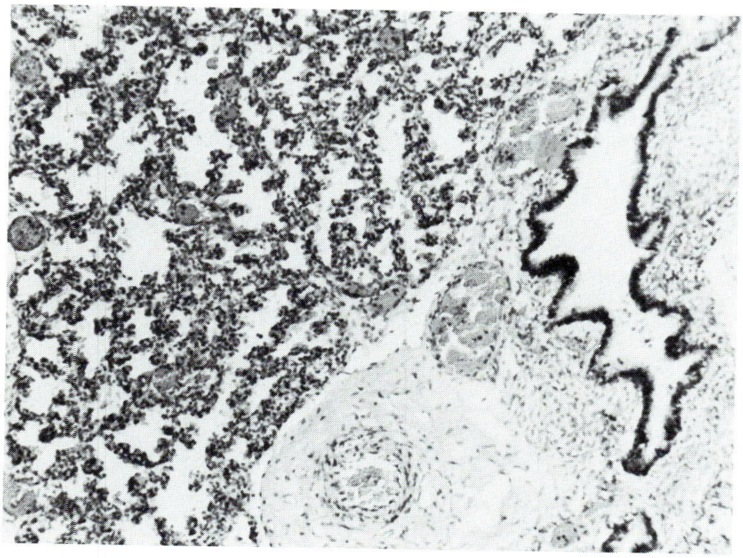

Figure 2–10. Lung hypoplasia in an infant with oligohydramnios. The lung is not adequately developed to allow for respiration.

5.2 PECTUS CARINATUM OR EXCAVATUM

GENESIS. Compression can alter the shape of the thoracic cage and result in depression or protrusion of the sternum.

FEATURES. Pectus excavatum (inward sternum), pectus carinatum (prominent sternum).

MANAGEMENT AND PROGNOSIS. In mild to moderately severe cases no management is usually utilized and the thoracic cage tends to improve with time. Surgical intervention merits consideration in severe cases for cosmetic reasons; it is unusual for such a deformity to affect respiration.

DIFFERENTIAL DIAGNOSIS. Thoracic deformities may occur concomitantly with abdominal muscle weakness, with a number of neurological disorders, with some skeletal dysplasias, and with a number of recognized syndromes.

A short chorda tendineae of the diaphragm may cause a pectus excavatum as may prolonged partial airway obstruction with inspiratory stridor.

5.3 SCOLIOSIS

GENESIS AND FEATURES. External constraint may cause scoliosis. To do so during late gestation, a fairly profound restraint, such as in a transverse lie, is necessary.

MANAGEMENT AND PROGNOSIS. Initial observation with manipulative stretching is merited in order to determine whether or not full reformation will occur after release from the presumed constraint. If there is not progressive improvement, successive bivalve plastic jackets should be made which tend to overcorrect the scoliotic bend.

DIFFERENTIAL DIAGNOSIS. Vertebral anomalies can result in scoliosis, as can neurological problems that alter muscle tone and some skeletal dysplasias.

6. NOSE DEFORMATION

GENESIS AND FEATURES. Small nose may result from compressive limitation of nasal growth in face presentation, and often is associated with transverse lie and with a small uterine cavity.

Compressed, downcurved nose is a feature of oligohydramnios and severe crowding, such as can occur in a bicornuate uterus.

Deviated nose is not rare and appears to be secondary to external constraint. The lower edge of the nasal cartilage may be dislocated from its placement on the vomerine ridge. This will result in an asymmetric nose with slanting of the columella and a smaller nasal aperture on the side toward which the cartilaginous septum is dislocated. About 2 per cent of newborn babies have an anterior dislocation of the nasal septum, and about 17 per cent have some septum deformation.

MANAGEMENT AND PROGNOSIS. The first two categories generally resolve spontaneously. The dislocated nasal septum should be treated about the third day after birth by repositioning the septal cartilage into the anatomical groove in the floor of the nose. The cartilaginous part of the nose is simply grasped between the thumb and forefinger, using gauze, and lifted forward while a probe or elevator is inserted into the nares below the free edge of the dislocated septum, forcing it into its normal location. A slight nasal asymmetry may persist for several weeks after relocation before the normal form is fully re-established. For the deformed septum that is not dislocated there is no known contraindication to manipulation to reposition the nose in an effort to restore the nasal septum to a normal alignment.

DIFFERENTIAL DIAGNOSIS. Small nose may be a feature in a number of specific disorders.

REFERENCES

1. Gray, L.P.: Septal and associated cranial birth deformities. Med. J. Aust. *1*:557, 1974.
2. Stoksted, P., and Schønsted-Madsen, U.: Traumatology of the newborn's nose. Rhinology *17*:77, 1979.

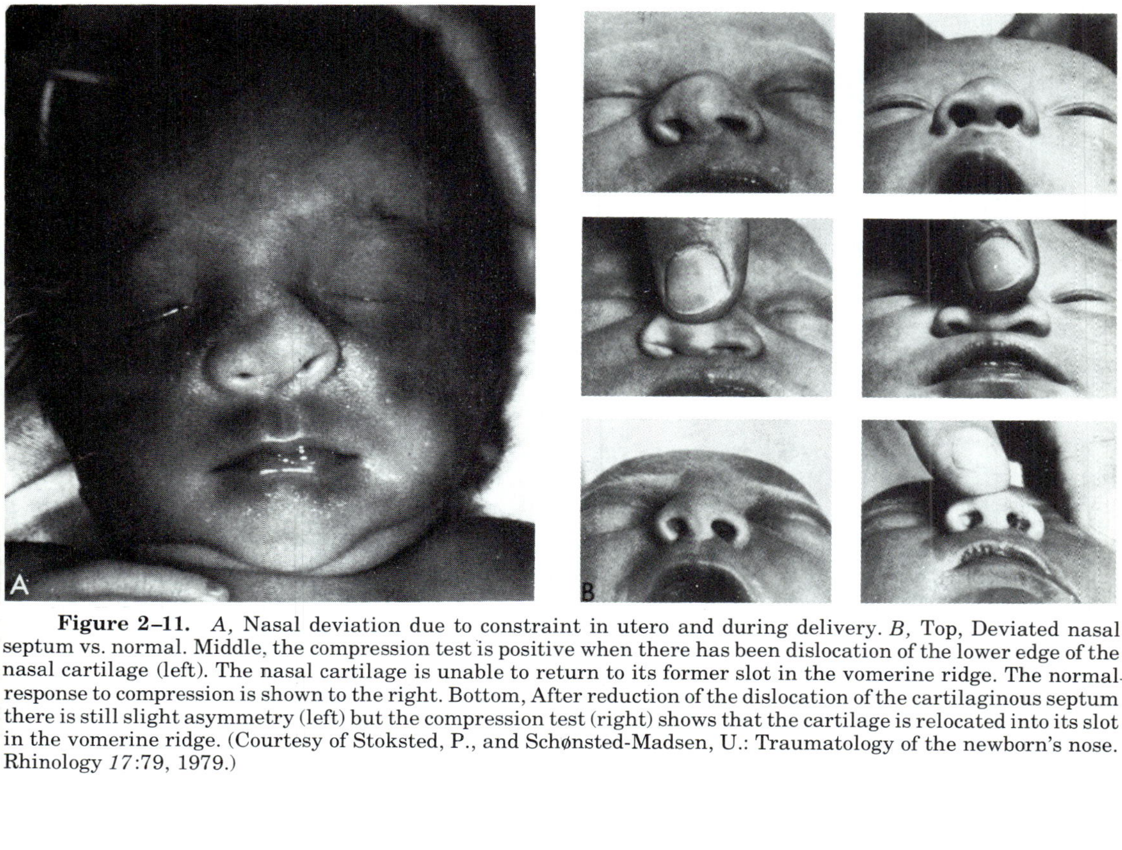

Figure 2–11. *A,* Nasal deviation due to constraint in utero and during delivery. *B,* Top, Deviated nasal septum vs. normal. Middle, the compression test is positive when there has been dislocation of the lower edge of the nasal cartilage (left). The nasal cartilage is unable to return to its former slot in the vomerine ridge. The normal response to compression is shown to the right. Bottom, After reduction of the dislocation of the cartilaginous septum there is still slight asymmetry (left) but the compression test (right) shows that the cartilage is relocated into its slot in the vomerine ridge. (Courtesy of Stoksted, P., and Schønsted-Madsen, U.: Traumatology of the newborn's nose. Rhinology *17*:79, 1979.)

7. EXTERNAL EARS

GENESIS AND FEATURES. *Accordion-type overfolding* of the upper helix and of other parts of the cartilaginous auricle is a frequent constraint deformity, as is *flattening of the ear against the head.*

Appearance of *low-set ear* may be engendered by molded skewing of the craniofacies, such as can occur with oligohydramnios or the constraint of a bicornuate uterus.

Finally, prolonged constraint of the external ear may result in *asymmetrical overgrowth* of the ear.

MANAGEMENT AND PROGNOSIS. Return toward normal from within the first few postnatal weeks tends to confirm the deformational origin of such ear defects, which generally require no management.

DIFFERENTIAL DIAGNOSIS. Aberrations of ear form caused by defects in development and/or function of auricular ear muscles, such as protruding auricle and lop ear, do not improve postnatally. A truly low-set ear is a very rare malformation.

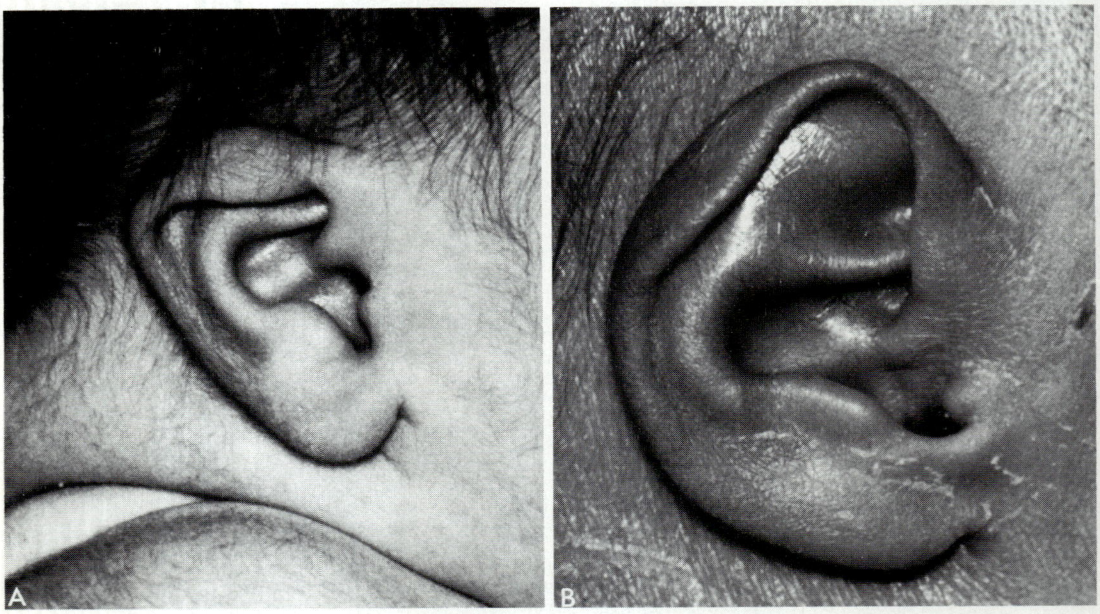

Figure 2–12. *A,* Constraint overfolding of scapha helix. *B,* Partial "crumpling" of ear form, especially concha.

Illustration continued on opposite page

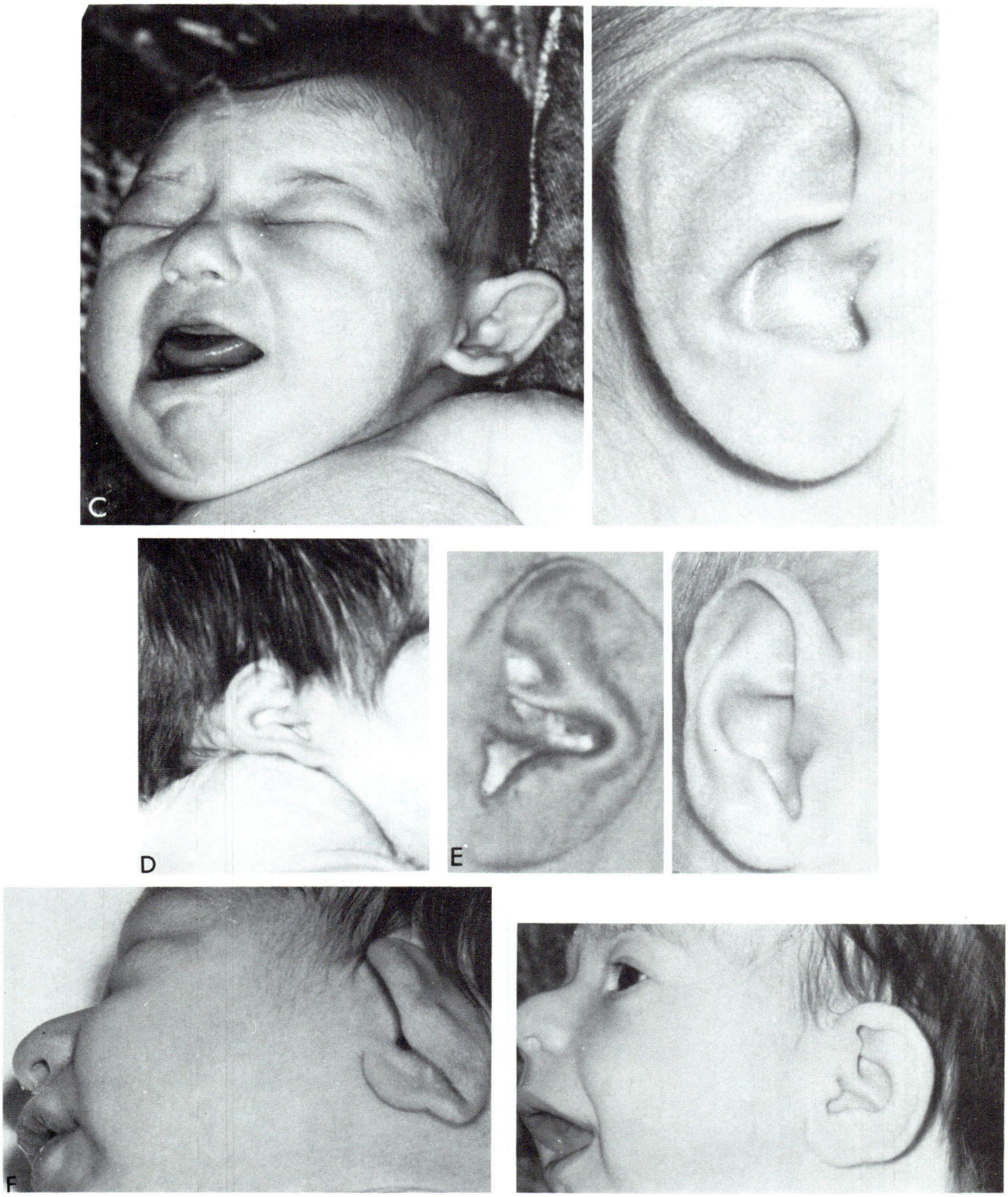

Figure 2–12 *Continued.* *C,* Uplifted crumpled ear caused by oblique skewed head position in utero, with the left auricle being caught between the shoulder and head (left), whereas the right ear was relatively flattened against the calvarium (right). *D,* Uplifted auricle caused by shoulder constraint under auricle in utero. *E,* Auricle flattened against head by oligohydramnios constraint at birth (left) and two months after being relieved from constraint (right). *F,* Left, Folded over auricle secondary to constraint in an asymmetric breech presentation in a septate uterus. Right, Twelve weeks later the auricle has largely returned to normal form. Taping the ear may accelerate the process of reformation.

8. MANDIBLE DEFORMATION

GENESIS AND FEATURES. *Micrognathia* may be caused by the chin being compressed against the chest. If the compression is of prolonged duration there may be a pressure indentation on the upper thoracic surface. Another cause is face presentation, with the mandible being a presenting part.

Mandibular asymmetry with a laterally tilted mandible is most commonly the result of the shoulder having been thrust up under the mandible in a breech presentation or in a prolonged vertex presentation.

MANAGEMENT AND PROGNOSIS. No management is usually required. Postnatally there is usually catch-up growth back to expected mandibular size and form.

DIFFERENTIAL DIAGNOSIS. There are a number of disorders in which micrognathia may be a feature. Asymmetrical mandible may occur with hemifacial microsomia.

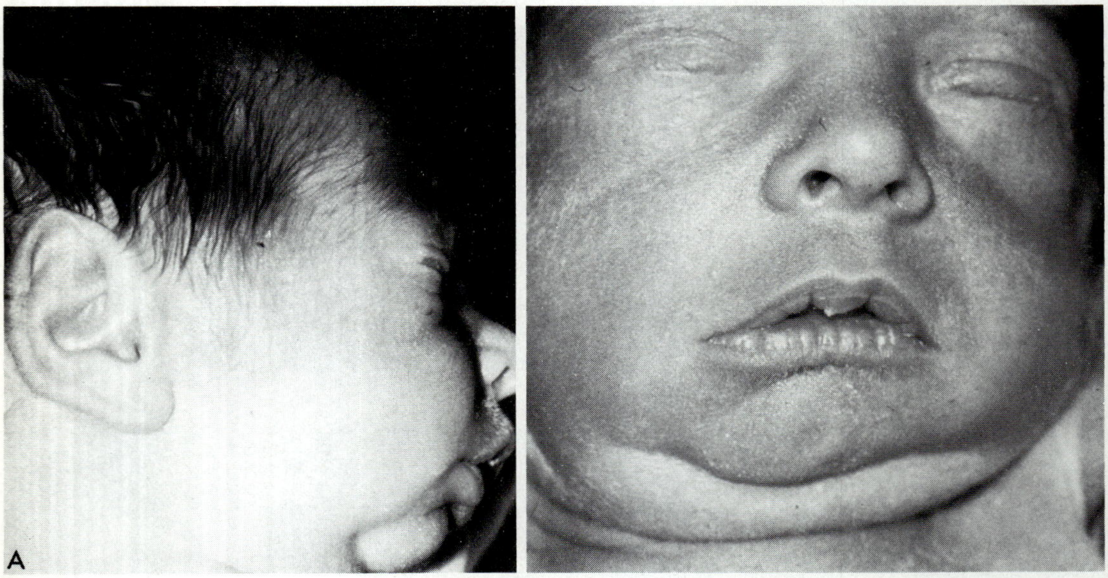

Figure 2–13. *A,* Micrognathia due to constraint. Note the redundancy of skin secondary to constraint-induced overgrowth of skin in the region.

Illustration continued on opposite page

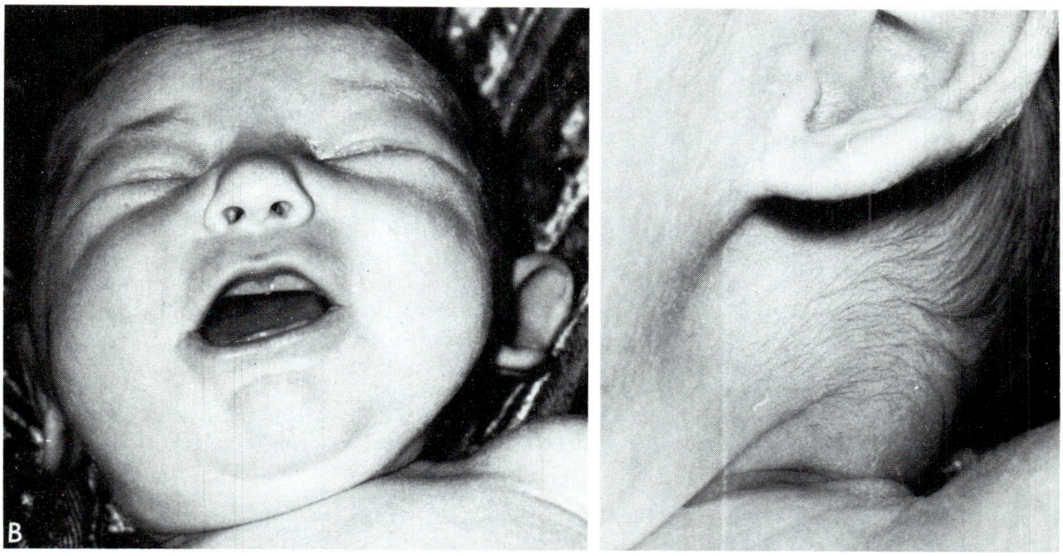

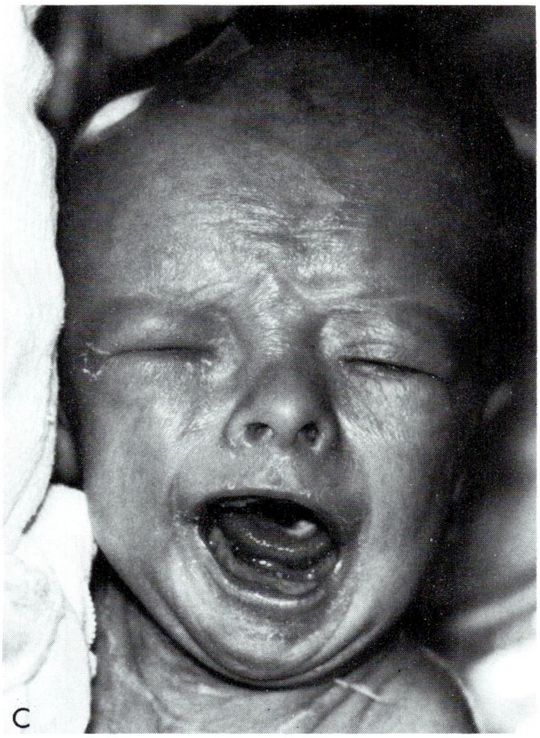

Figure 2–13 *Continued.* *B*, Mandibular asymmetry with sloping angulation of alveolar ridge secondary to unilateral shoulder compression. Note the sulcus impression made by the shoulder (right). *C*, Marked asymmetry secondary to unilateral shoulder compression in utero.

9. STERNOCLEIDOMASTOID TORTICOLLIS

GENESIS AND FEATURES. Prenatally acquired torticollis usually occurs in conjunction with the obliquely shaped plagiocephalic head in response to the head being caught askew. One hypothesis is that the constraint on the side of the neck causes ischemic changes in the middle portion of the sternocleidomastoid muscle, with secondary fibrosis and sometimes a palpable fusiform fibrous mass, the sternocleidomastoid "tumor." The shortening of the muscles tends to maintain the aberrant posture of the head and face with the head tilted toward the affected side and the chin rotated toward the opposite, unaffected convex side, the "side facing the sun." Persistence of the torticollis may result in continued facial asymmetry, even to the degree that the eyes are at different levels.

MANAGEMENT AND PROGNOSIS. Mild degrees of torticollis improve spontaneously, especially those without a palpable fusiform fibrous "tumor." Neck stretching is recommended. More rigorous modes of management are set forth under plagiocephaly (disorder number 10).

DIFFERENTIAL DIAGNOSIS. Disruptive tearing of the sternocleidomastoid muscle may occur at birth, especially during the delivery of the aftercoming head in vaginal breech delivery.

REFERENCE

1. Clark, R.N.: Diagnosis and management of torticollis. Pediat. Ann. *5*:43, 1976.

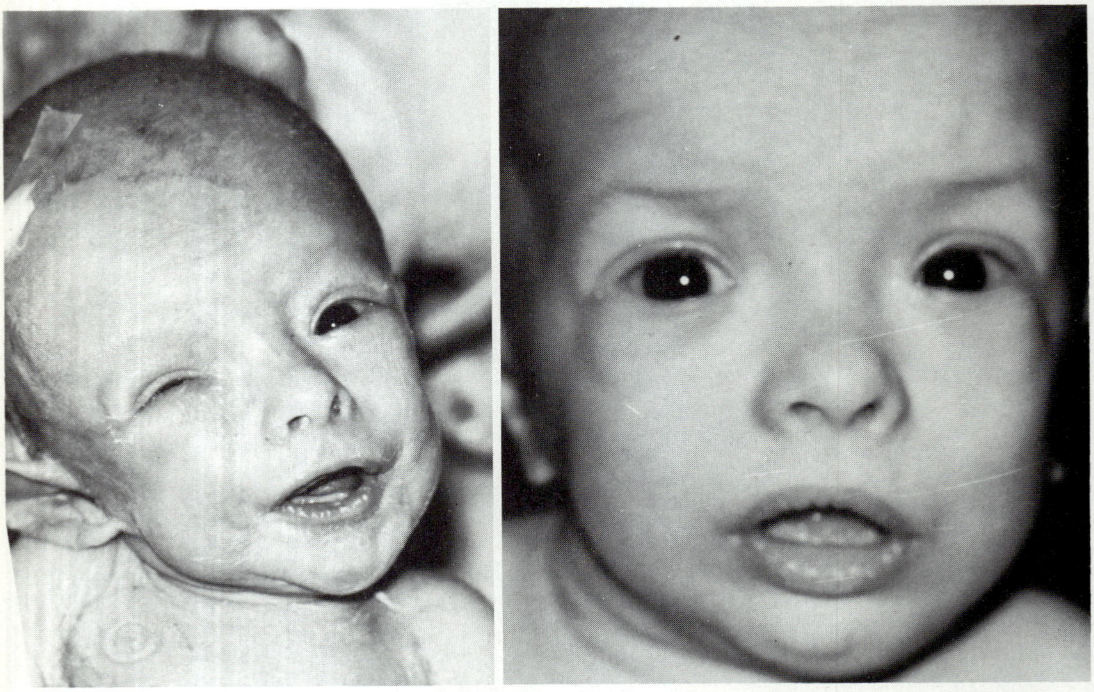

Figure 2–14. Torticollis with shortening of the right sternocleidomastoid muscle as part of the impact of the head being compressed askew onto the right shoulder (left). With conservative stretching, the face was almost symmetrical by several months of age (right).

10. OBLIQUE HEAD DEFORMATION — PLAGIOCEPHALY-TORTICOLLIS SEQUENCE

GENESIS. During late fetal life the head may tend to be compressed to one side. Such obliquity of forces usually results in asymmetrical molding of the craniofacies. The same compression may have an adverse effect on the sternocleidomastoid muscle, resulting in ischemic changes in the middle portion of the muscle without consequent fibrosis and torticollis. Lop-sided head constraint is most likely to occur in first-born babies and in larger babies. The deformations are more commonly left sided, possibly on the same proposed basis as for left-sided predilection for dislocation of the hip: namely, the propensity of the fetus to lie with its left side toward the mother's back.

FEATURES

Craniofacial and Neck. Oblique molding of the head yields asymmetrical prominence of the side of the forehead that is tilted downward, with contralateral prominence of the occiput. The degree of craniofacial distortion may be sufficient to cause a variant placement of the eyes. The external ear on the compressed side has often been partially folded or thrust out by the compression of the shoulder. The mandible will often be asymmetrical and tilted. Scoliosis may be present, as may other deformities such as dislocation of the hip. The position of comfort is with the head tilted to one side and the neck in the torticollis position. If there has been damage to the sternocleidomastoid muscle on the side that was held askew, this situation may tend to perpetuate the torticollis positioning. The asymmetrical craniofacies fosters the tendency of the infant to lie on one side of the head or face, in the position of comfort, and thus maintain the deformity.

MANAGEMENT, PROGNOSIS, AND COUNSEL. In most instances of plagiocephaly with torticollis it would seem reasonable to observe the infant during the first two to three months after birth in order to determine whether spontaneous resolution will take place. During this conservative period of observation there are a few procedures that might be worth utilizing. The surface upon which the baby's head rests should be relatively soft, the infant's crib should be placed so that attractive objects such as people and mobiles are on the side away from the torticollis, and the head and neck may be moderately overstretched away from the torticollis several times a day. Another measure that can be utilized is to place a silk or nylon stocking of the proper size to fit snugly, but not tightly, over the baby's calvarium. The lower part of the stocking is tied into a knot, and the stocking is cut and fitted in such a manner that the knot tends to force the baby to lie on the more prominent side and thus avoid perpetuating the deformity. I learned this technique from a physician whose name I unfortunately do not recall. If little or no improvement has occurred by two to three months of age, a more rigorous form of management should be considered.

One relatively conservative mode of management is the construction of a helmet that will restrain growth at the prominent parts of the head but allow the shallow parts of the head to grow. Thus the prominent parts are restrained while brain growth provides the mechanical forces from within to force out the shallow regions of the calvarium. The method begins by making a plaster cast of the infant's deformed head. The cast is cut off, taped together again, and filled with modeling clay or other material, such as plaster, and the cast is removed. Material is then added to the model where the head is shallow, but none is added where the head is unduly prominent. Thus a more ideally shaped head is modeled. From the new model, a fiberglass or plastic helmet is made, much like an American football helmet. It is tight where the infant's head is prominent and allows for growth in the less prominent regions. Once brain growth has filled out the helmet, no further management is usually needed. If the torticollis persists after the helmet is utilized for several weeks, then rubber straps may be placed from the helmet to the sides of the crib at night in such a manner as to force the infant to hold the head toward the side opposite the favored one. If the helmet constraint therapy is utilized by two to four months of age, it usually requires only two to three months to re-form the head to a more normal shape. However, if the helmet management is not employed until seven to eight months, it may require four to five months to achieve the desired result. The pace of re-formation relates to the rate of brain growth, which is much more rapid during the first six months than later in infancy.

Other modes of management that have been utilized include resection of the sternocleidomastoid muscle. This may be considered in the second or third year if the foregoing measures have not been successful. Hopefully the more conservative helmet form of management will obviate the need for this procedure.

The majority of mild to moderately severe instances of plagiocephaly with torticollis improve to normal spontaneously.

DIFFERENTIAL DIAGNOSIS. A malformation of the cervical vertebrae may be the primary cause of the head being askew, in which case the deformation of plagiocephaly and torticollis would be secondary to an intrinsic malformation problem. In such relatively rare instances the response to the foregoing modes of management would not be expected to be as favorable as for an external constraint deformation.

A neuromuscular disorder may be the primary cause of the head being askew; in such instances the prognosis would be again relatively poor.

Asymmetric craniostenosis of coronal or lambdoidal sutures may produce an asymmetric head. However, it is usually possible to distinguish constraint deformation from craniostenosis by the prenatal history, clinical appearance, palpation of the suture lines, and the natural history after birth — without utilizing roentgenography or other studies.

Postnatally, neuromuscular disorders, particularly those predisposing toward hypotonia, and occasionally severe neglect may cause an infant to lie in a particular position for a prolonged period of time, long enough to give rise to asymmetric molding of the head. This can usually be distinguished from congenital constraint plagiocephaly by the history at birth and the natural history after birth.

Prematurely born infants usually have poor muscle tone and relatively malleable heads. If they persistently lie on a firm surface toward one side of the head there may be postnatal development of plagiocephaly. Again this may be distinguished from postnatal constraint deformation by the history.

REFERENCES

1. Clarren, S.K., Smith, D.W., and Hanson, J.W.: Helmet treatment for plagiocephaly and congenital muscular torticollis. J. Pediatr. *94*:43, 1979.
2. Jones, P.G.: Torticollis in Infancy and Childhood. Sternomastoid Fibrosis and the Sternomastoid "Tumour." Springfield, Ill., Charles C Thomas, 1968.
3. von Reuss, A.R.: The Diseases of the Newborn. New York, William Wood and Co., 1921.

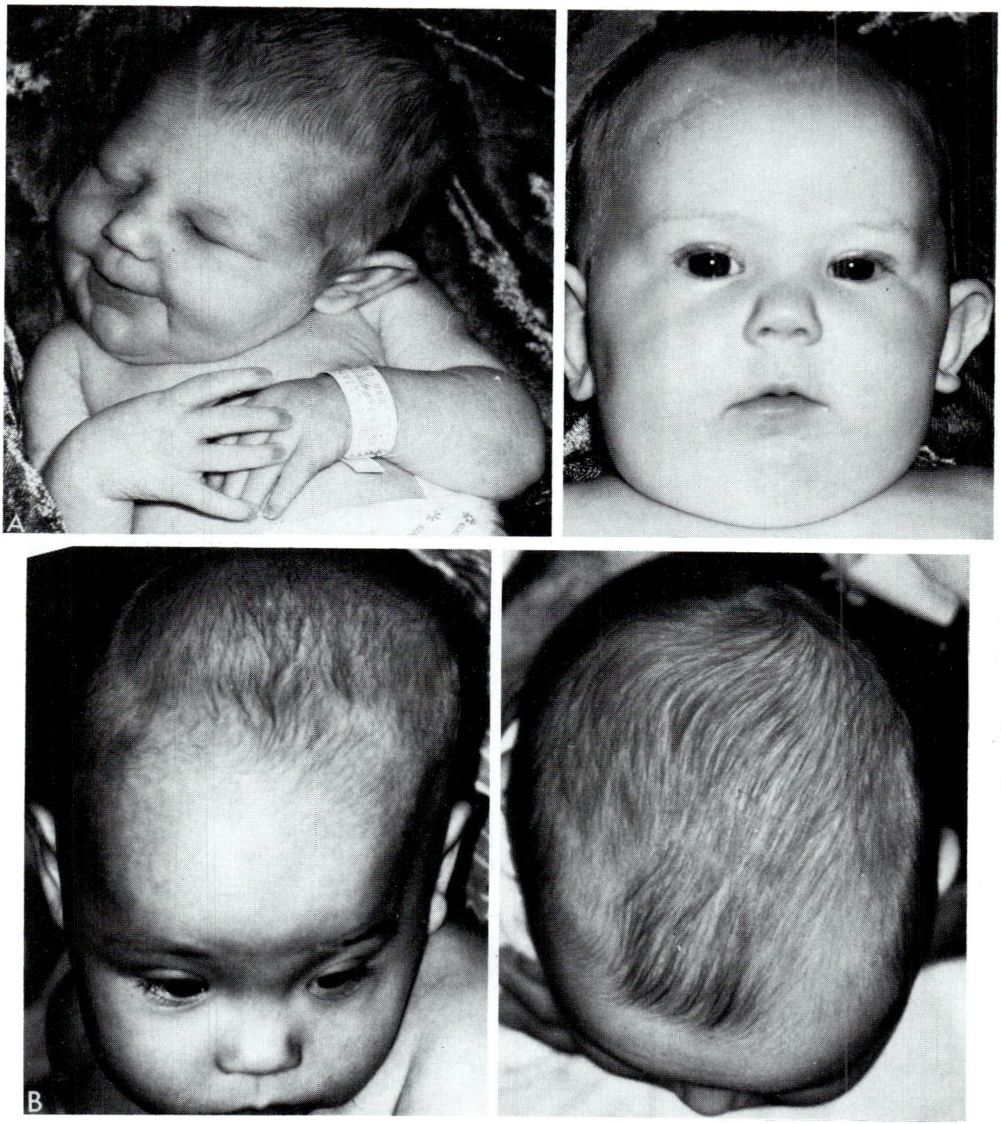

Figure 2–15. *A,* Left, "position of comfort" of a large baby who had been in an oblique presentation for some weeks before delivery, yielding the lopsided head with torticollis. Right, same baby at five months of age showing marked improvement from manipulation alone. The auricle, though improved, is still moderately deformed. *B,* Varying degrees of oblique-shaped plagiocephalic heads in two young infants.

Illustration continued on following page

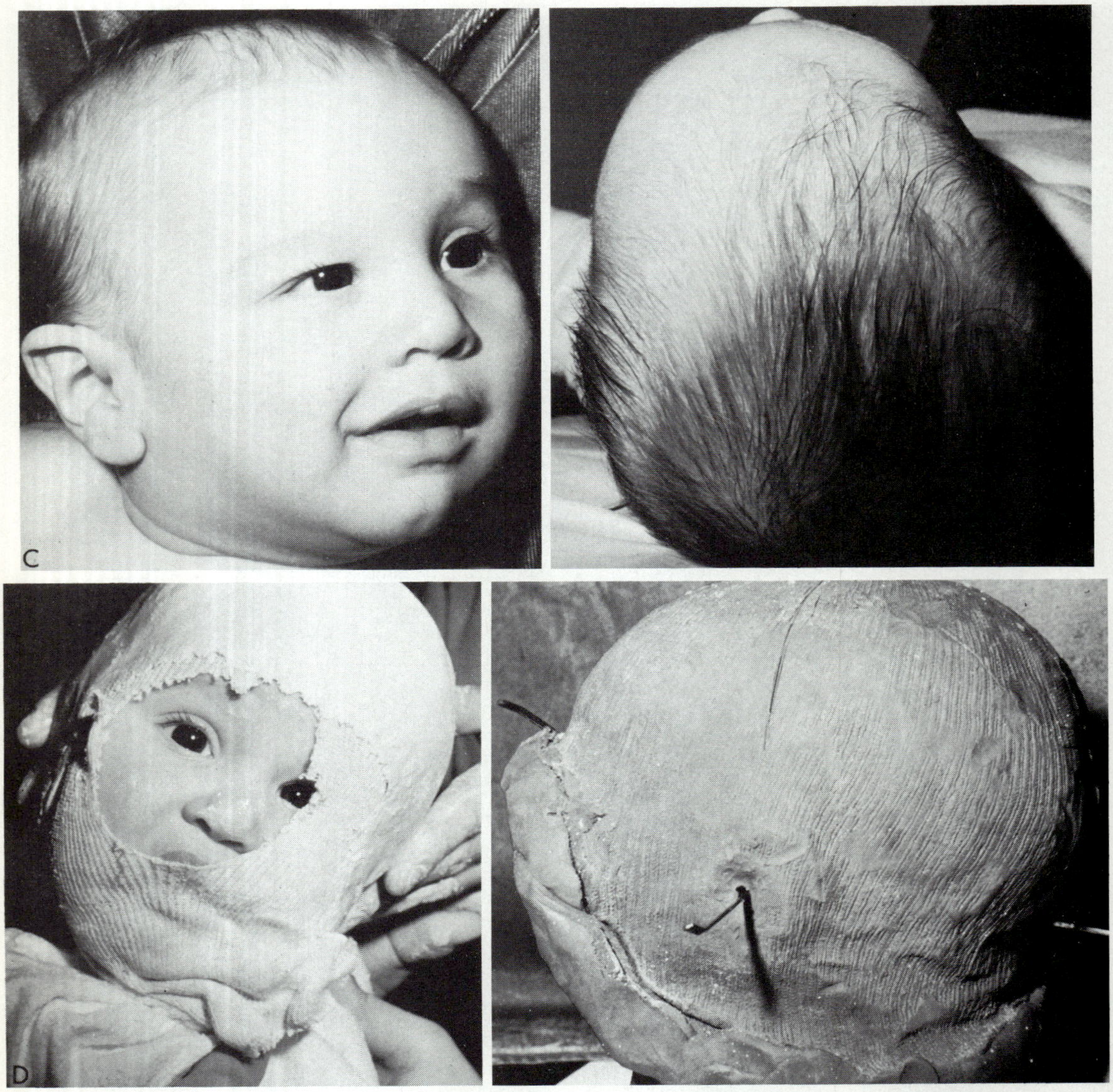

Figure 2–15 *Continued.* *C,* Four-month-old infant with plagiocephaly and torticollis for whom more conservative measures had not been successful. Therefore, a helmet was made, as shown in *D* and *E*. *D,* In order to make the helmet, a plaster cast is made of the head shape. The mother is asked to leave the room when the cast is "buzzed" off. The form of the cast is now filled with modeling clay, though more recently plaster of paris has been utilized. The bobby pins mark the ear, nose, and occipital prominence landmarks. The model is then sculptured by adding clay (or plaster of paris) to the shallow areas, leaving the full prominent regions alone.

Illustration continued on opposite page

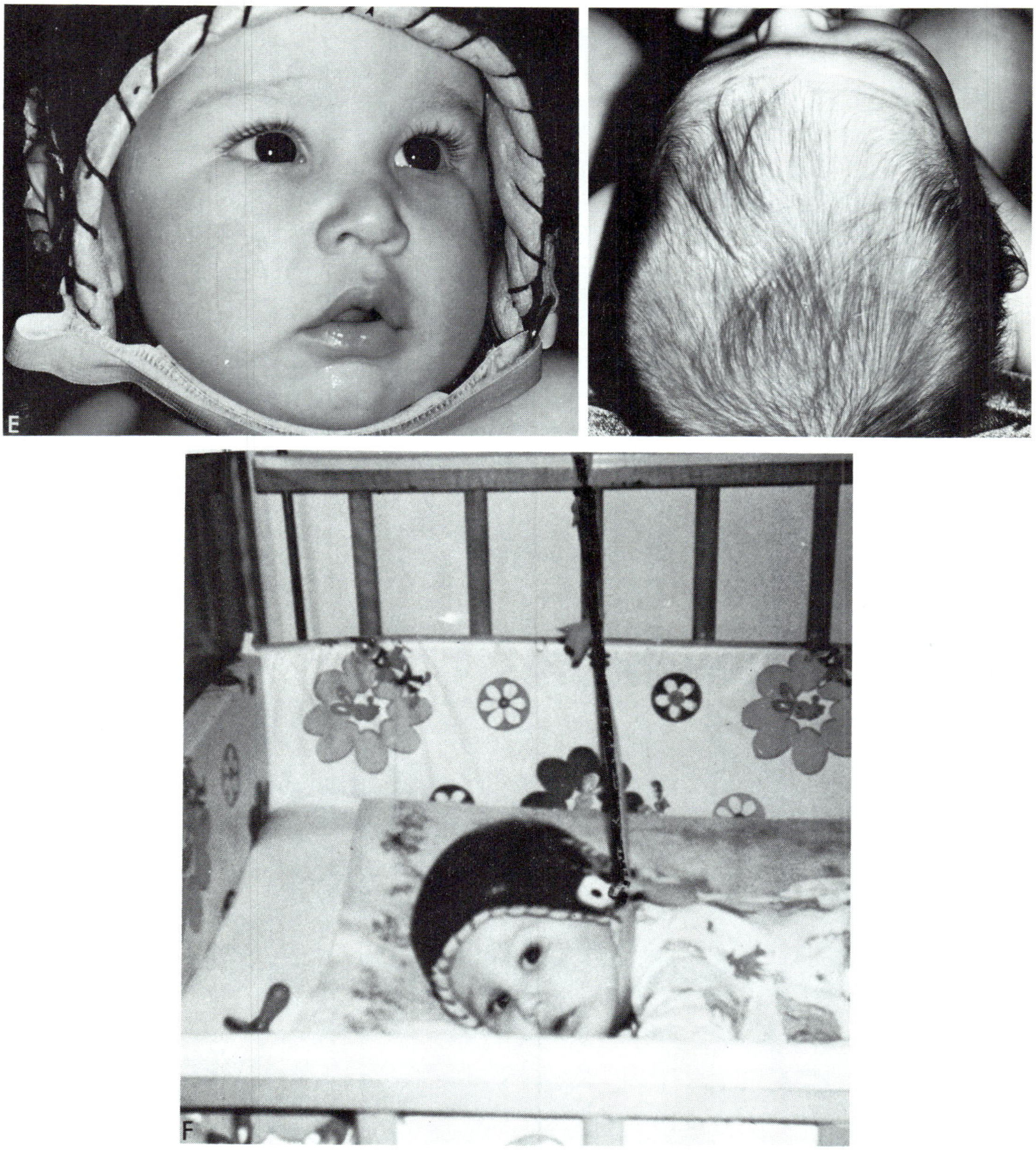

Figure 2–15 *Continued.* *E,* A helmet is then made over the more normally contoured model. This one was made with fiberglass. Dr. Sterling Clarren now utilizes plastic. Most prosthetic shops would be able to make such a helmet. It is now tight where the infant's head was full and allows for growth (via brain growth) in the shallow regions. The liner and chinstrap provide a close facsimile to an American football helmet. This lad "filled out" the helmet between four and six months, by which time his head and face were reasonably symmetrical. (From Clarren, S. K., Smith, D. W., and Hanson, J. A.: Helmet treatment for plagiocephaly and congenital muscular torticollis. J. Pediatr. *94*:43, 1979.) *F,* The torticollis persisted in the above infant after the helmet was initially placed on his head. Therefore, rubber straps (shown in back) were attached to the sides of his helmet in his crib at night; these stretched his head to the opposite side. If he tried to resume his old torticollis position, "whingo!", his head would swing to the corrective side. After seven to ten days the torticollis was resolved.

Illustration continued on following page

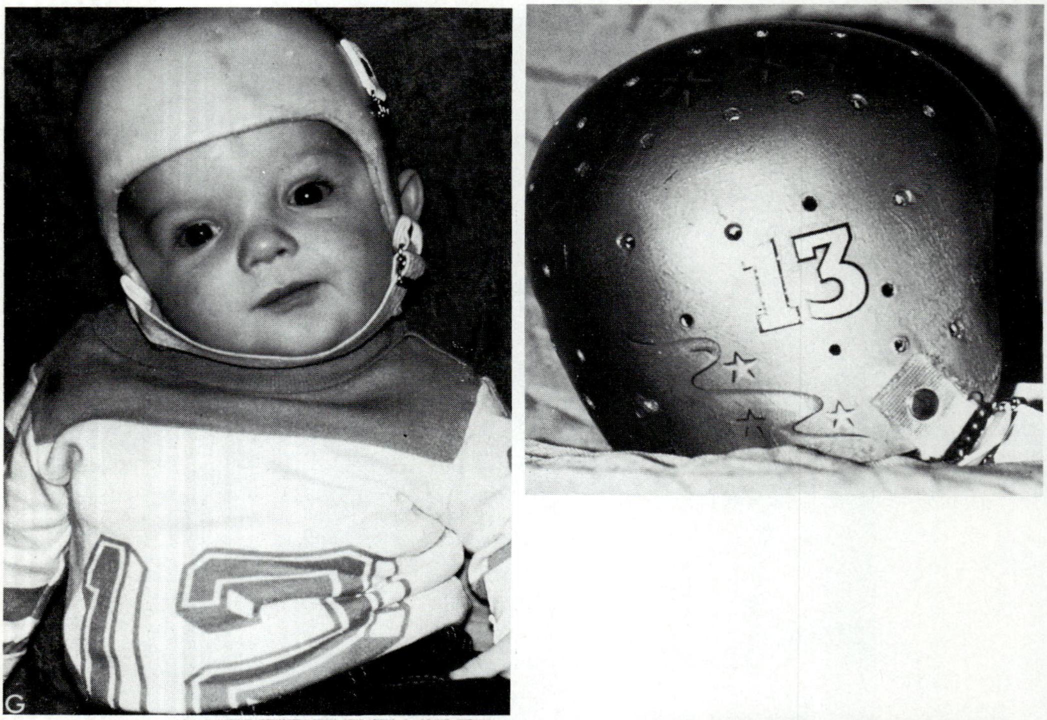

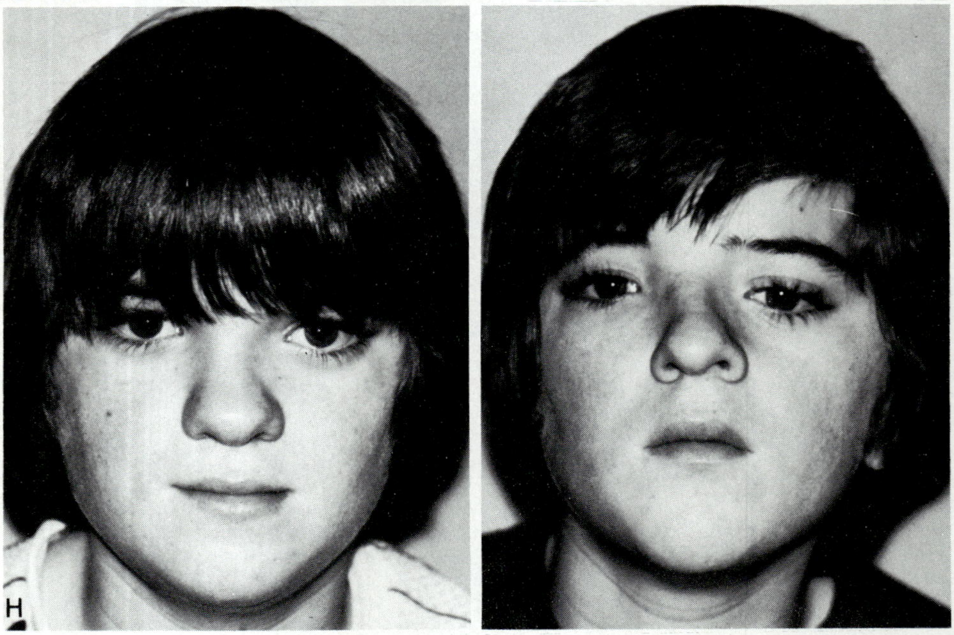

Figure 2–15 *Continued. G,* We supply the helmets, but the rest is supplied by the parents of these future football players of America! *H,* Although most mild degrees of plagiocephaly with torticollis will resolve spontaneously, permanent deformation can result, as shown in these 10-year-old monozygotic twins who are not "identical" because one incurred a greater degree of in-utero head molding than the other.

11.0 CRANIOSTENOSIS, GENERAL

GENESIS. Limitation of the normal growth stretch at a suture during fetal life may result in craniostenosis. This has been shown to occur, for example, when the lack of growth stretch is caused by a deficit in brain growth, as in severe primary microcephaly. Experimental sutural immobilization through application of glue to young rabbit sutures has been shown to result in secondary craniosynostosis at the site of the growth restriction of the suture.[1] The most common cause of craniostenosis in the human is considered to be constraint of the fetal head in utero.[2-4] The external constraint limits growth stretch in the direction between the constraining points and may cause craniostenosis of an intervening suture. The constrained suture tends to develop a bony ridge, especially at the point of maximal constraint. This will prevent future growth at that site, and the expanding brain will then distort the calvarium into aberrant shape.

FEATURES. The features are dependent on which sutures are stenotic, the extent of craniostenosis, and the timing of the problem. The earlier the craniostenosis occurs, the more profound is its impact on subsequent craniofacial and brain development. Craniostenosis of both the sagittal and coronal sutures, with or without involvement of other sutures, may limit overall brain growth and result in increased intracranial

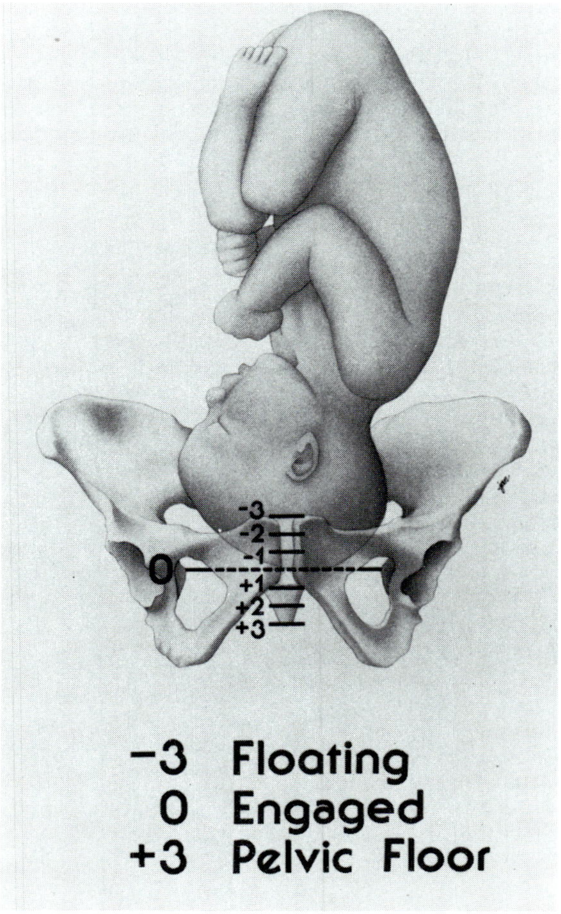

Figure 2–16. Craniostenosis, general. The head may become engaged in the pelvis in such a manner as to limit lateral growth at the sagittal suture. This is considered to be a factor that can enhance the risk of sagittal craniostenosis. (Courtesy of Jan A. Norbisrath, Medical Illustrator, Obstetrics and Gynecology, University of Washington Medical School.)

pressure. On roentgenogram, the cranial vault, which is under increased pressure because of craniostenosis, tends to have a "beaten silver" appearance. The precise reason for this phenomenon is not known, but it may be the result of altered magnitude and direction of forces on the bony trabecular organization within the calvarium.

MANAGEMENT AND PROGNOSIS. Mild degrees of craniostenosis may not merit treatment. However, in moderate to severe cases, early surgical therapy is usually warranted. Except for instances in which both the coronal and sagittal sutures are stenotic, impairing brain growth, the predominant indication for surgery is cosmetic restoration toward normalcy. Martin P. Sayers,[5] a pediatric neurosurgeon with extensive experience with the problem of craniostenosis, states: "I've never had a family complain about the surgical result, but we've had bitter recriminations about non-operative results." The surgical approach pioneered by Dr. Sayers,[5] at Columbus Children's Hospital in Ohio, involves removing the aberrant portion of the bony calvarium from its underlying dura, including the area of the stenotic suture(s). If this is done within the first few months after birth a new bony calvarium will usually develop within the remaining dura mater under the same principles that normally guide calvarial morphogenesis;[6] namely, that intradural mineralization begins between the sites of dural reflection. As long as there is continued growth stretch from the expanding brain, the sites over the dural reflections remain unossified, thereby forming the sutures. Thus the calvarium and its sutures may develop normally after a partial calvariectomy for constraint-induced craniostenosis. The new bony calvarium begins to develop within two to three weeks and is usually firm by five to eight weeks. If the procedure is done after three to four months of age, the approach is similar with the exception that pieces of the calvarium are replaced in a mosaic over the dura mater in order to act as niduses for mineralization of the new calvarium.

DIFFERENTIAL DIAGNOSIS. There are a number of other causes for craniostenosis.[7] These can be divided into several general categories such as problems of the brain or mesenchymal tissues and metabolic disorders.

Brain Problems. Basic problems in early brain morphogenesis may cause a lack of dural reflection and hence lack of a suture and, thereby, inability of the calvarium to grow laterally in that region.[6] Observed examples include: (1) holoprosencephaly (single ventricle) with no anterior interhemispheral fissure and consequently no metopic suture; (2) unilateral deficiency of the early cerebrum with no insular sulcus and hence no sphenoid wing or its dural reflection and thus no coronal suture. Deficit of brain growth, such as in severe microcephaly, may result in a lack of expansile brain force with craniostenosis as a secondary consequence. More localized brain growth deficiency may cause a particular suture to become prematurely craniostenotic. For example, frontal brain growth deficiency may result in metopic craniostenosis. Excessive shunting of hydrocephalus may also cause a lack of growth stretch at the suture lines, enhancing the liability toward craniostenosis.

Mesenchymal Tissue Problems. There are a number of disorders in which craniostenosis appears to occur because of an aberration in mesenchymal tissues. One such example, Apert syndrome, features not only craniostenosis but also osseous syndactyly. Most of these disorders are genetically determined.

Metabolic Problems. Early rickets, regardless of its cause, is strangely liable to result in craniosynostosis. In rare instances early hyperthyroidism also has been a cause, as has hypercalcemia.

REFERENCES

1. Persing, J.A., and Jane, J.A.: University of Virginia Medical School, personal communication.
2. Graham, J.M., Jr., deSaxe, M., and Smith, D.W.: Sagittal craniostenosis: Fetal head constraint as one possible cause. J. Pediatr. *95*:747, 1979.
3. Graham, J.M., Jr., Badura, R., and Smith, D.W.: Coronal craniostenosis: Fetal head constraint as one possible cause. Pediatrics *65*:995, 1980.
4. Graham, J.M., Jr., and Smith, D.W.: Metopic craniostenosis and fetal head constraint: Two interesting experiments of nature. Pediatrics, *65*: 1000, 1980.
5. Sayers, M.P.: Columbus Children's Hospital, Columbus, Ohio. Personal communication.
6. Smith, D.W., and Töndury, G.: Origins of the calvarium and its sutures. Am. J. Dis. Child. *132*:662, 1978.
7. Freeman, J.M., and Borkowf, S.: Craniostenosis: Review of the literature and report of thirty-four cases. Pediatrics *30*:57, 1962.
8. Hanson, J.W., Sayers, J.P., Knopp, L.M., Macdonald, C., and Smith, D.W.: Total neonatal calvariectomy for severe craniosynostosis. J. Pediatr. *91*:257, 1977.

CRANIOSTENOSIS

11.1 CRANIOSTENOSIS, SAGITTAL

GENESIS. Early descent of the fetal head into the maternal pelvis, often four weeks or more before delivery, with entrapment and biparietal constraint is considered the most common cause of sagittal craniostenosis.[2] This mode of genesis is shown in Figure 2–17*A*. The sagittal ridging tends to be most prominent at the site between the parietal eminences, the position of greatest theoretical lateral constraint. The platypelloid pelvis, relatively small in the anterior-posterior when compared with the lateral dimensions, would hypothetically constitute the greatest risk for this type of entrapment head constraint. Sagittal craniostenosis is the most common type of craniostenosis, occurring about once in 2000 births. It has a 3:1 predilection for males. This has been attributed to the more rapid rate of head growth in the male during the last trimester of gestation.[2] The larger head is simply more likely to become seriously constrained.

FEATURES. The head is long and narrow with a prominent forehead and occiput. There is a ridge along the mid to posterior sagittal suture which is most prominent at the biparietal diameter. The relatively excessive anterior-posterior growth may partially spread the coronal and/or lambdoidal sutures.

The head circumference may be spuriously increased, providing a mistaken impression of macrocephaly or even hydrocephaly.

MANAGEMENT, PROGNOSIS AND COUNSEL. (See also the section on general craniostenosis.) Craniostenosis of the sagittal suture alone imposes a moderate cosmetic problem. It may sometimes be difficult for the parents and physician to resolve the question as to whether or not surgical intervention is indicated. One woman who never had surgery experienced severe pressure-type headaches at 13 to 15 years of age. In retrospect, these were interpreted as having been secondary to increased intracranial pressure during her adolescent brain growth spurt at a time when the other sutures were unable to completely accommodate to the problem of the sagittal craniostenosis.

Partial calvariectomy should include all of the sagittal suture region and a wide zone to either side. For the best cosmetic results, the bony calvarium of the occipital and bregmal promontories may be excised; these promontories will not recur.

Most constraint-induced instances of sagittal craniostenosis are sporadic; however, it has not been determined whether some of the rather rare instances of familial sagittal craniostenosis are of this type, are a consequence of inherited pelvic type, or are part of a broader pattern of malformation.

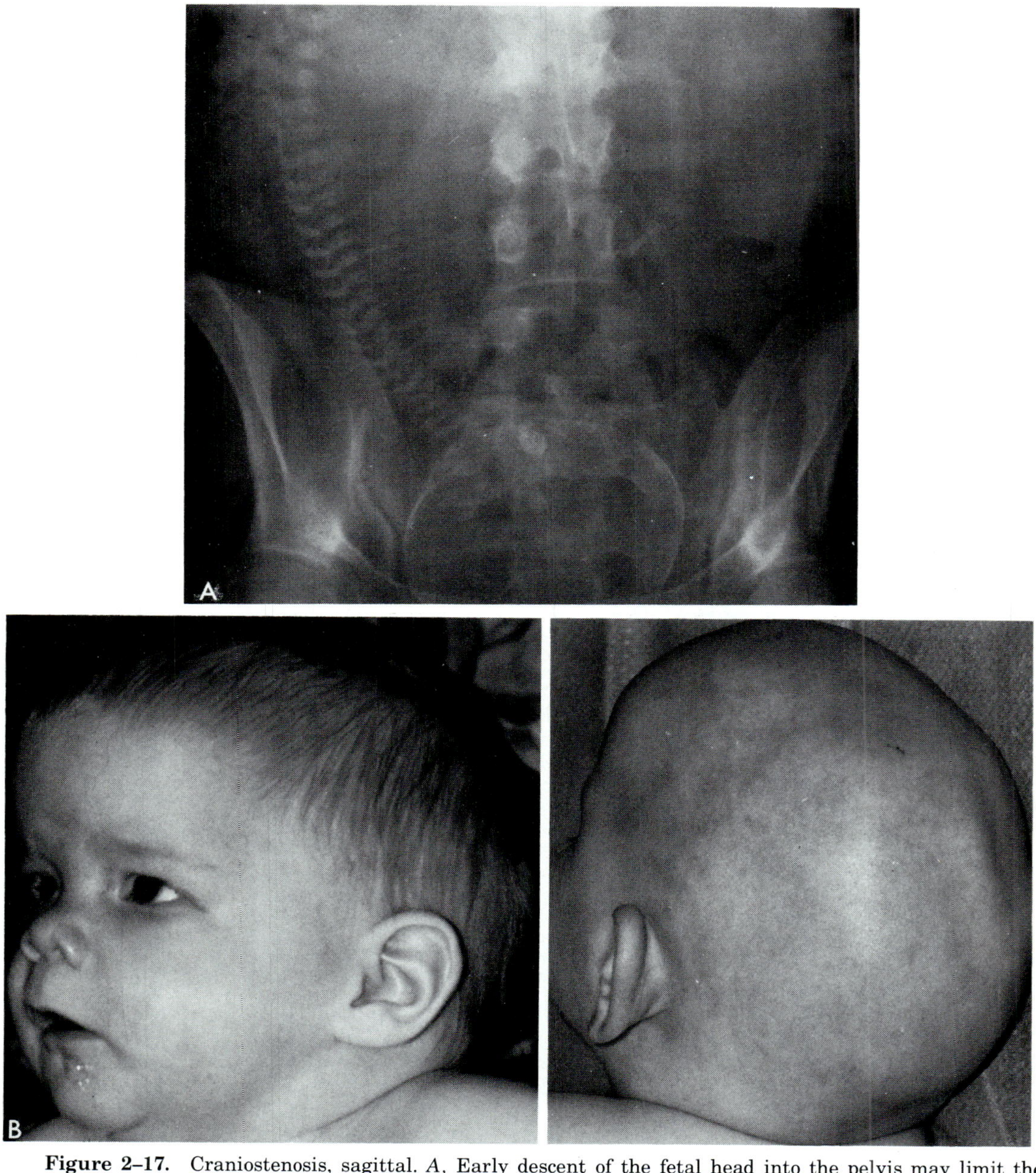

Figure 2–17. Craniostenosis, sagittal. *A,* Early descent of the fetal head into the pelvis may limit the lateral growth stretch at the sagittal suture line, resulting in craniostenosis. The roentgenogram shows the engaged fetal head of an infant who was noted to have sagittal craniostenosis at birth. *B,* Infant with sagittal craniostenosis. Note the prominent forehead with the scaphocephalic head. Ridging of the sagittal suture was most prominently evident at the area between the biparietal sites of presumed in-utero constraint of lateral head growth.

Illustration continued on following page

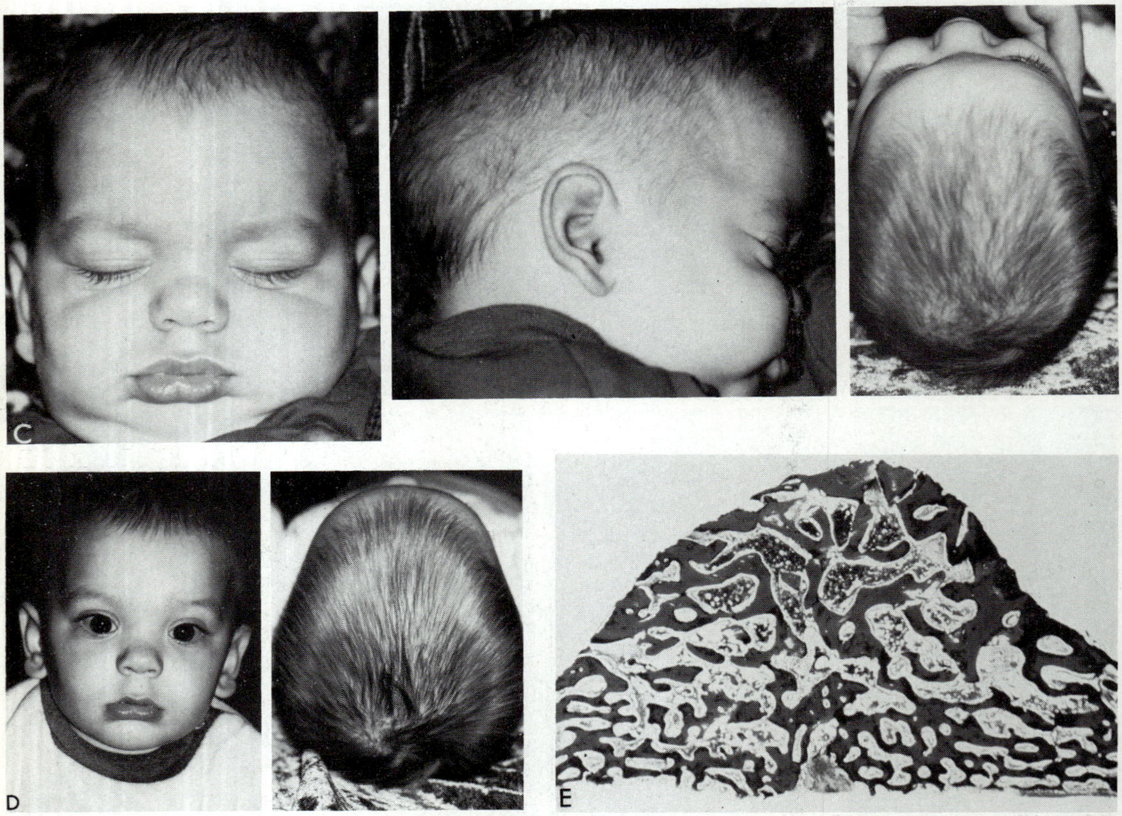

Figure 2–17 *Continued.* *C,* Infant with sagittal craniostenosis. Note the relatively narrow biparietal diameter of the scaphocephalic head. *D,* Above infant at nine months of age following partial calvariectomy with correction of sagittal craniostenosis. Note the dramatic change in the bifrontal versus biparietal dimensions in the top view of the head. *E,* Histology shows ridged synostotic suture with resorption of bone at inner table of the calvarium at the site between the usual parietal eminences.

Illustration continued on opposite page

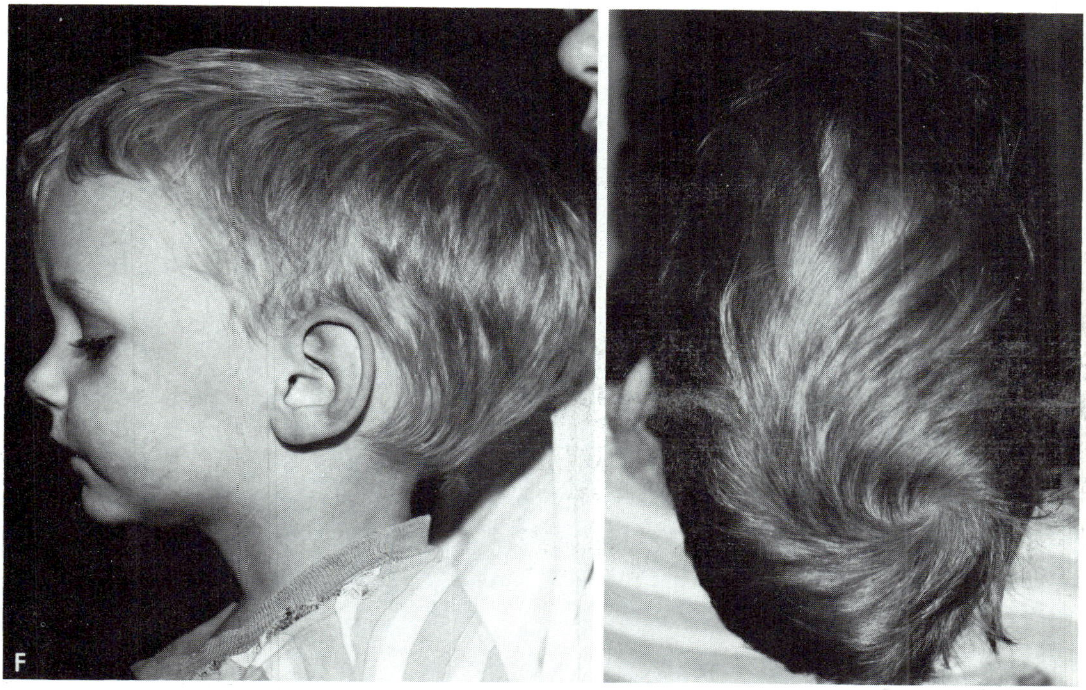

Figure 2–17 *Continued.* *F,* Six year old with unoperated sagittal craniostenosis.

11.2 CRANIOSTENOSIS, CORONAL

GENESIS. Constraint-induced coronal craniostenosis has been considered to be secondary to early descent of the fetal head into a constraining pelvis, to aberrant fetal lies, and to bicornuate uterus.[3] The left side is more commonly affected than the right, and this has been ascribed to the LOA birth position, which tends to result in more coronal constraint on the left side than on the right.[3] The coronal stenosis secondarily affects the anterior craniofacies, as is shown in Figure 2–18*A*.

FEATURES. The suture area is usually ridged, and the head is short and wide. The impact of the coronal stenosis on the craniofacies is summarized in Figure 2–18*A*. When it is unilateral, the impact on the facies is unilateral and the face may be quite asymmetrical. Within the skull the sphenoid ridge tends to be high and thin.

MANAGEMENT, PROGNOSIS, AND COUNSEL. The cosmetic impact of coronal craniostenosis is of such magnitude that early surgical intervention is generally warranted. Furthermore, the child with untreated coronal stenosis has a small nasopharynx that tends to foster middle ear infection and an oral situation that contributes to both speech problems and dental malocclusion. The partial calvariectomy for coronal stenosis should start behind the area of the coronal suture and extend well below the suture laterally. Sayers[5] also recommends removal of the bony sphenoid ridges as far medially as is feasible. The bony resection should be extended frontally to include the brow and the orbital roofs (prior to four months of age). The brain may then move forward and model the new anterior calvalrium. Furthermore, the cranial base, which is the roof of the face, can grow forward and carry the midface with it. Thus, the secondary craniofacial aspects of coronal craniostenosis can be largely re-formed toward genetic expectation. However, in order to accomplish this, the surgery should ideally be done in early infancy. The forward growth of the cranial base is 56 per cent complete by birth and 70 per cent complete by two years of age.

DIFFERENTIAL DIAGNOSIS. The sequence of coronal synostosis may occur by itself or (in the author's experience) as a rare autosomal dominant disorder usually referred to as Crouzon syndrome. It may also occur in a number of syndromes, such as Apert syndrome and Saethre-Chotzen syndrome, in which other features such as syndactyly are present.

Constraint limitation of craniofacial growth may occasionally yield an appearance at birth which is quite similar to that of coronal stenosis and its consequences, *without* craniosynostosis being found at the time of early surgery. Such patients demonstrate rapid spontaneous restitution toward normal form in the first few postnatal weeks, which would not be expected with coronal stenosis. For this one reason it is probably best to wait several weeks or longer before making a decision as to calvarial surgery, unless the problem is severe with evidence of increased intracranial pressure.

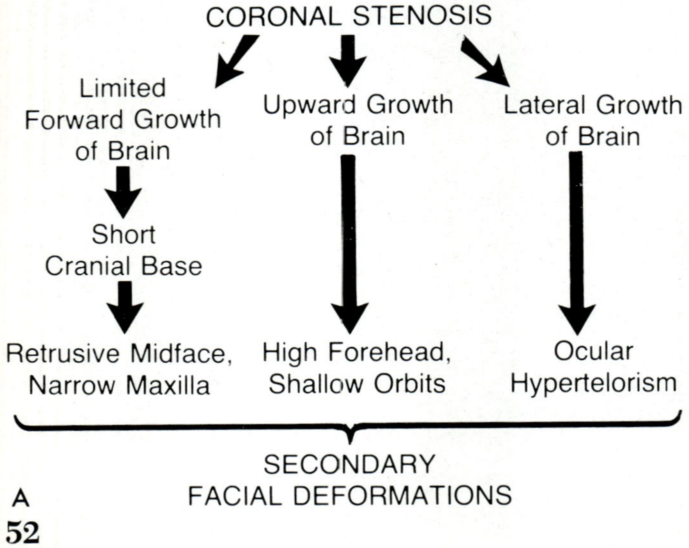

Figure 2–18. Craniostenosis, coronal. *A*, Coronal craniostenosis in early life appears to result in secondary facial deformations.

Illustration continued on opposite page

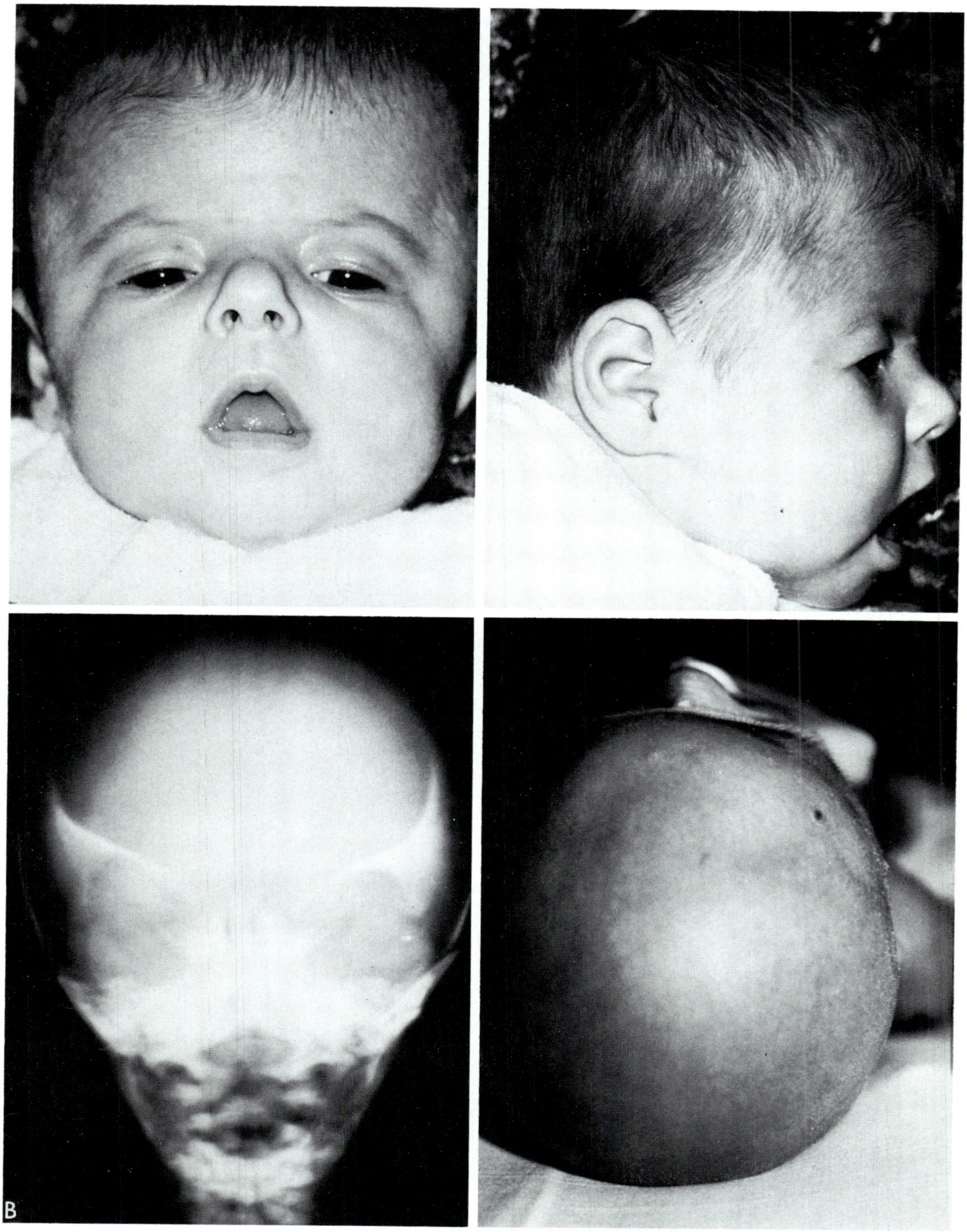

Figure 2–18 *Continued.* *B*, Bilateral coronal craniostenosis interpreted as being due to intrauterine constraint in a young infant with secondary facial deformations, short brachycephalic head, and "harlequin" radiographic sign caused by upward flare of the sphenoidal ridges.

Illustration continued on following page

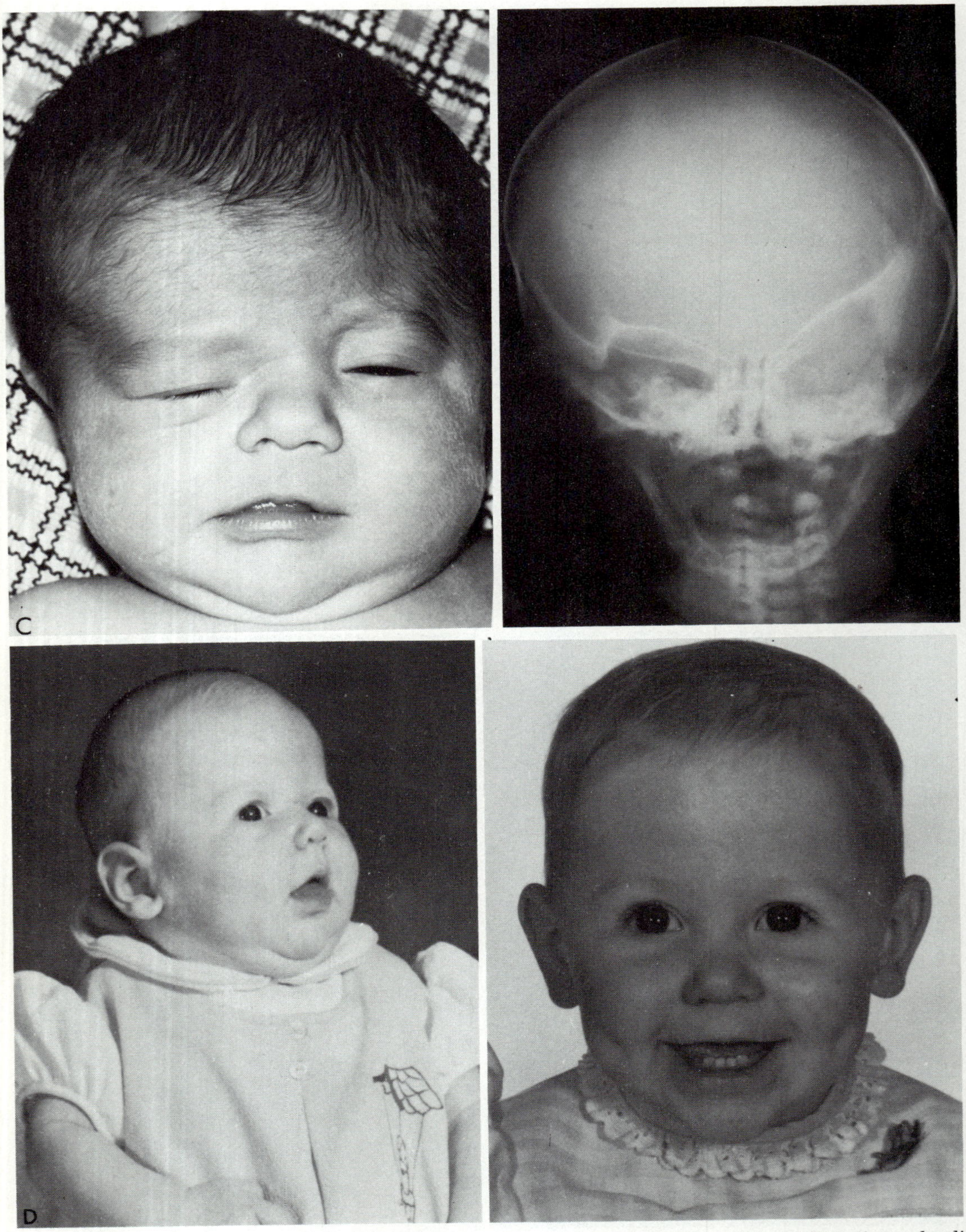

Figure 2–18 *Continued.* *C,* Unilateral coronal craniostenosis yielding unilateral facial distortion and radiographic harlequin sign. *D,* Early surgical intervention at several months (left) of the coronal craniostenosis (by Dr. Nelson) allowed the mid-face to move forward to yield a normal facies by 14 months (right).

11.3 CRANIOSTENOSIS: SAGITTAL PLUS CORONAL

GENESIS. Constraint as the causation of sagittal plus coronal sutures is unusual and would usually be of profound degree.

FEATURES. In this condition the limitations of calvarial expansion are so severe that there is limited room for brain growth. Besides the oxycephalic head shape with the coronal stenosis impact on the craniofacies, usually there are signs of increased intracranial pressure and a "beaten silver" roentgenographic appearance of the inner table of the skull. There may also be optic atrophy, proptosis, and loss of vision.

MANAGEMENT, PROGNOSIS. Early extensive calvariectomy is merited to preserve brain function and development as well as to allow for re-formation of the craniofacial skeletal features.

DIFFERENTIAL DIAGNOSIS. This degree of craniostenosis is more commonly found in some of the genetically determined disorders, such as Apert syndrome and Saethre-Chotzen syndrome.

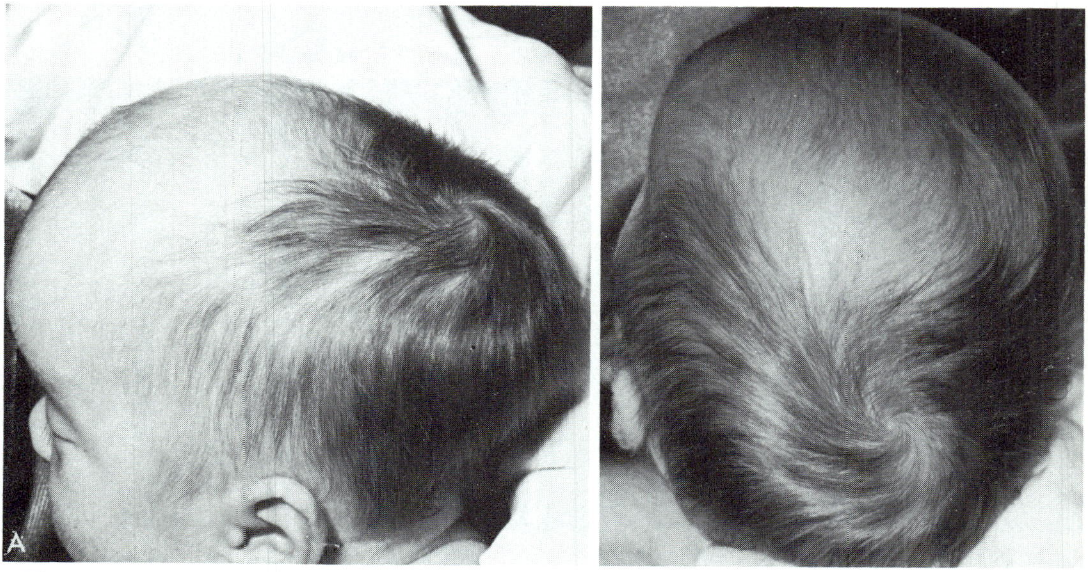

Figure 2–19. Craniostenosis, sagittal plus coronal. *A,* Three-week-old infant with sagittal, coronal, and lambdoidal craniosynostosis. Only the metopic suture was open and the brain growth ballooned out into this region, which was under increased pressure. The coronal synostosis plus the bulging forehead region had distorted the mid and upper facies. A calvariectomy was performed by Dr. Peter Sayers from the supraorbital ridge to below the coronal suture, above the mastoid and above the foramen magnum. The aberrant calvarium was discarded, and within several weeks a new calvarium was forming from the remaining dura mater.

Illustration continued on following page

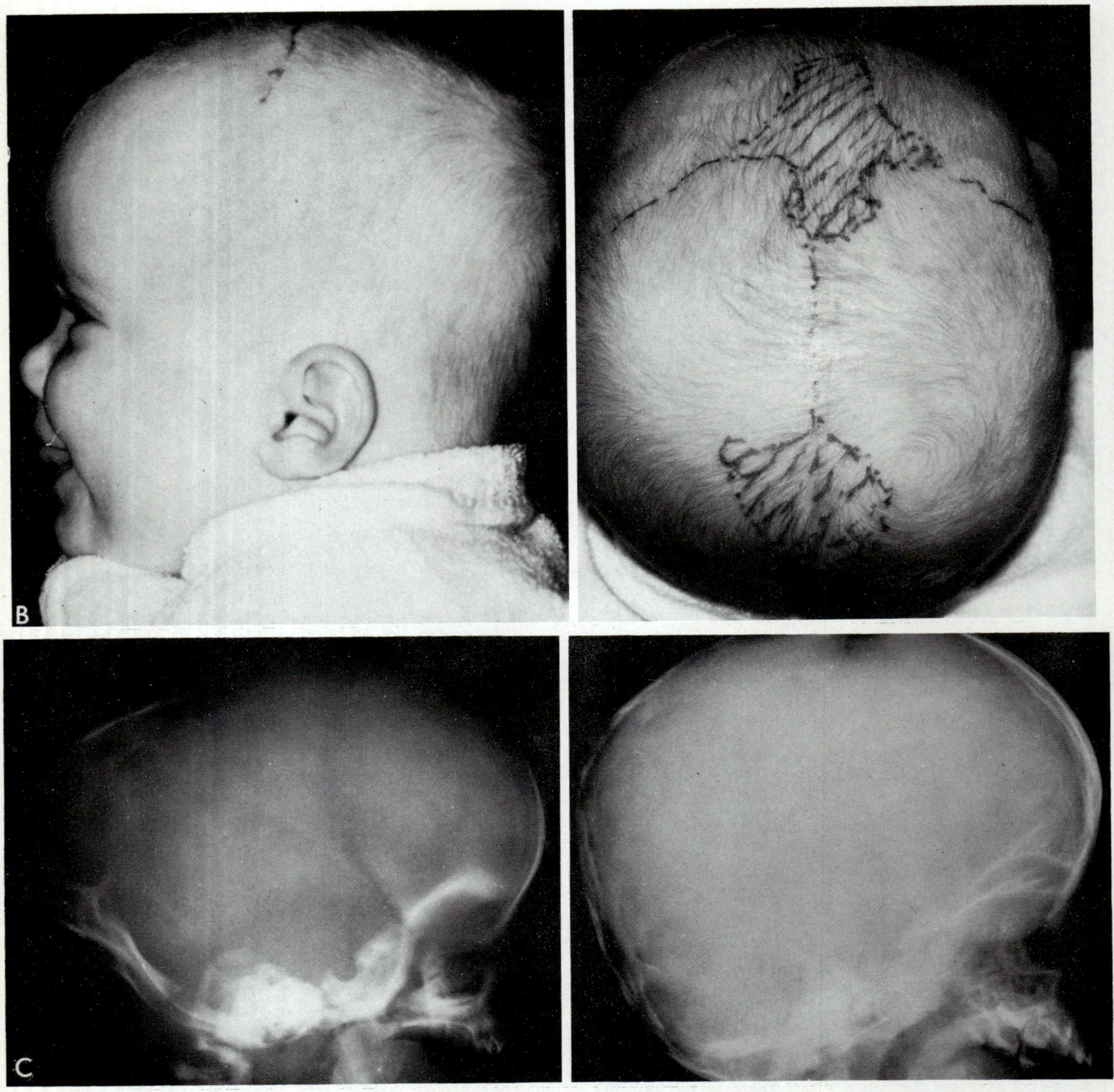

Figure 2–19 *Continued. B,* The infant in *A* two months after calvariectomy. The brain of normal size and shape has been the guiding force in the shape of the upper head as the new calvarium has formed. The new calvarium has functional sutures at the sites of dural reflection and fontanels where the sutures join. *C*, Radiograph of the above infant before calvariectomy and after the new calvarium has formed. (*A, B,* and *C* are from Hanson, J. W., Sayer, M. P., Knopp, L. M., Macdonald, C., and Smith, D. W.: Subtotal neonatal calvariectomy for severe craniosynostosis. J. Pediatr. *91*:257–260, 1977.)

11.4 CRANIOSTENOSIS, METOPIC

GENESIS. Lateral constraint of the frontal part of the head may cause early metopic craniostenosis.[3] Examples have included one of MZ triplets whose forehead had been wedged between the buttocks of her two sisters in utero and an infant whose head had been "impacted" in a bicornuate uterine horn.

FEATURES. A narrow and sometimes prow-shaped forehead with a ridged metopic suture. There may be secondary upslanting to the palpebral fissures and ocular hypotelorism.

MANAGEMENT AND PROGNOSIS. Generally no treatment is utilized in mild cases. Moderate to severe instances often warrant a frontal calvariectomy, ideally including the entire forehead down to the supraorbital ridges. In the more severe cases that include hypotelorism the brows and orbital roofs should also be removed.

DIFFERENTIAL DIAGNOSIS. It is important to exclude primary defects of brain, such as the holoprosencephaly malformation complex.

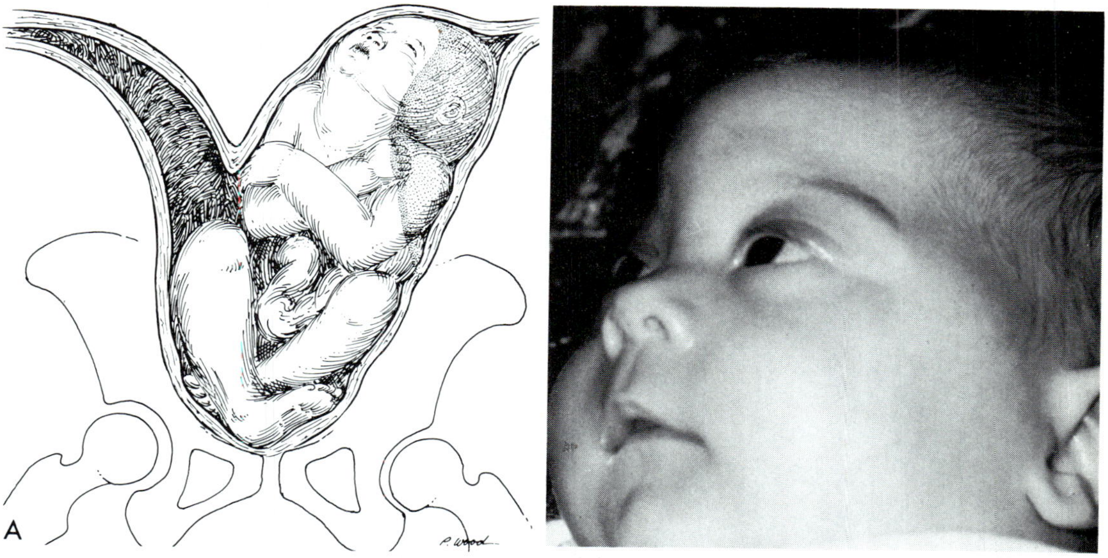

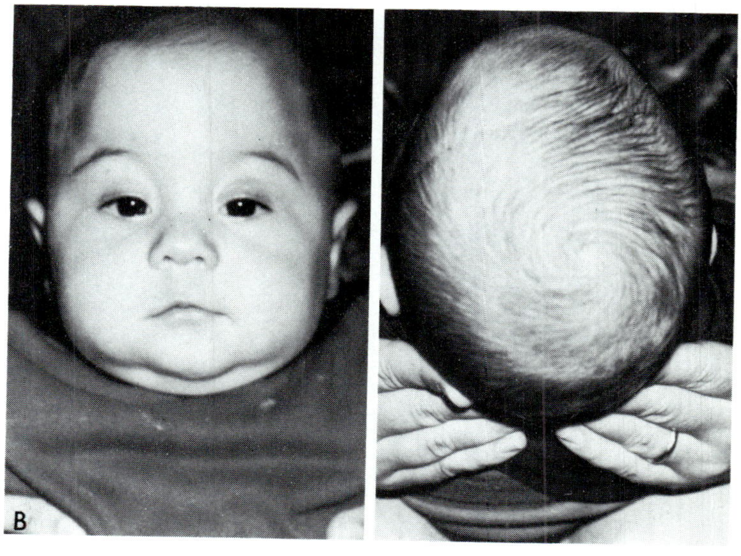

Figure 2–20. Craniostenosis, metopic. *A,* Metopic craniostenosis in an infant who was reared in a bicornuate uterus. At cesarean section it required several minutes to dislodge the head from its tightly entrapped position in one upper uterine horn. *B,* Postoperative status of the infant shown in *A* following calvariectomy of the frontal bone region down to the supraorbital ridges, allowing the brain to remold the forehead as a more normally shaped bony calvarium was formed.

Illustration continued on following page

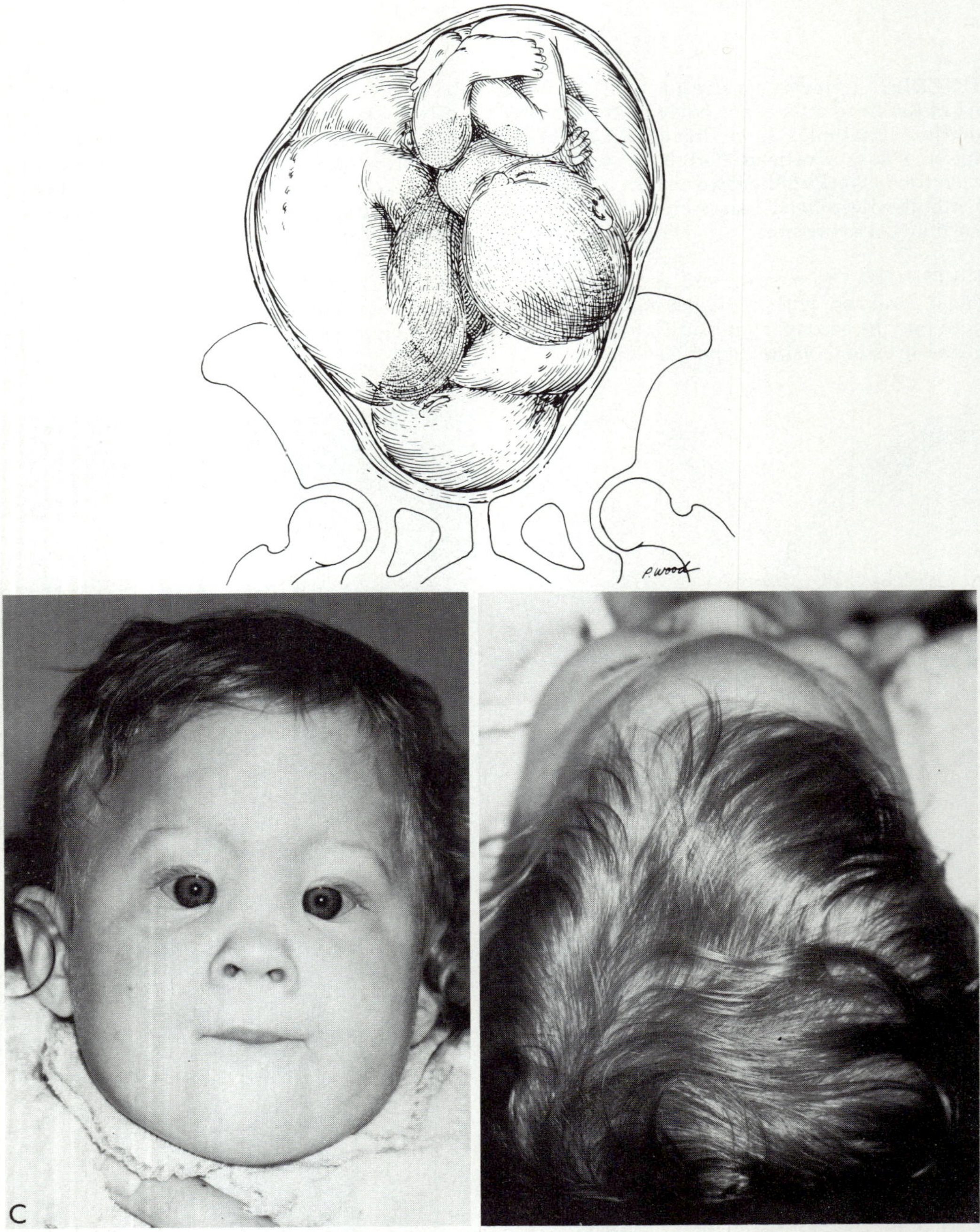

Figure 2–20 *Continued.* *C,* One of monozygotic triplets reared in a 104 pound woman who gained 64 pounds during the pregnancy. Roentgenograms had shown the patient (upper left in in-utero illustration) to have the frontal portion of her head wedged between the buttocks of her co-twins. This was considered the source of the constraint that yielded the metopic craniostenosis with secondary narrow forehead and upslanting palpebral fissures, features which were not shared by her monozygotic co-twin.

11.5 CRANIOSTENOSIS, LAMBDOIDAL

Craniostenosis of the lambdoidal suture is rather unusual. Whether fetal head constraint may cause this problem remains to be determined; we have not had an opportunity to study such cases since this mode of etiology was implicated.

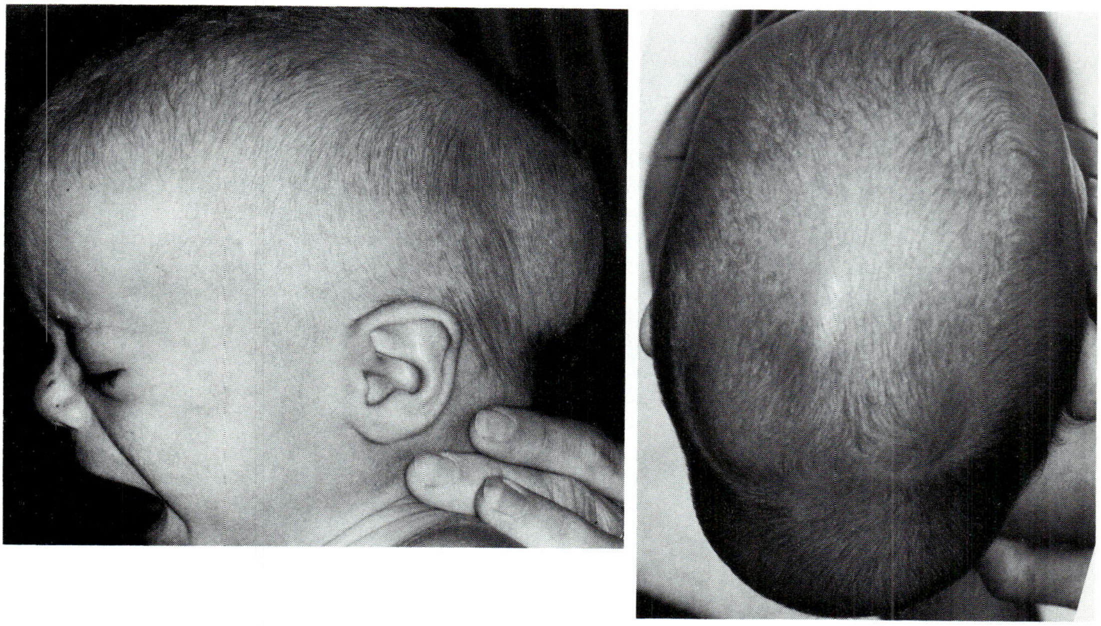

Figure 2–21. Craniostenosis, lambdoidal. Prominent occiputal bulge in an infant who has both lambdoidal and posterior sagittal craniostenosis, with palpable ridging at the sites of craniostenosis.

12. VERTEX BIRTH MOLDING

GENESIS. In the normal fetus presenting in the vertex position there may be appreciable molding of the head at birth, especially if he or she is the first born or is a large baby or if the mother has a prolonged labor, has a small pelvic outlet, and/or has an incompletely dilated rigid cervix.

The following is a tentative reconstruction of how the molding normally occurs. During the initial cervical dilation there is some decrease in the biparietal diameter, with a prominence and increased height of the vertex. With incomplete cervical dilation the biparietal diameter is decreased further and there is increasing angulation toward the presenting part. The occipital bone rotates inward on the "occipital hinge," and the frontal bones bend inward. The result is a decrease in the anterior-posterior diameter.

FEATURES. The forehead tends to slope and the parieto-occipital region is prominent. Overlapping at sagittal, coronal, and/or lambdoidal sutures is frequent. Head circumference measurements may be spuriously low because of the nature of the molding. The head circumference may shift upward by one to three days after birth as the head remolds in relation to the true brain shape. The head usually shifts back to the original unmolded form by six days after birth.

Occasionally there may be a traumatic subperiosteal hemorrhage, most commonly in the outer table of the parietal bone. This will give rise to a soft, fluctuant circular mass. With time its borders will become elevated and crater-like, as the raised periosteum begins to deposit bone at its borders. At the leading part of the parieto-occipital region there may be edema of the skin and subcutaneous tissues, the so-called caput succedaneum.

Hemorrhages may occasionally be evident in the sclerae and in the retina.

PROGNOSIS. The prognosis for spontaneous resolution of the vertex birth molding and the traumatic components that may accompany it is generally excellent and no therapy is necessary other than reassurance that the baby is normal.

DIFFERENTIAL DIAGNOSIS. A spuriously small occipitofrontal head circumference may give a mistaken impression of varying degrees of microcephaly, as may the sloping forehead. Clinical judgment as to the apparent overall brain size plus follow-up head circumference measurement as the calvarium returns toward a normal shape will usually resolve any questions in this regard.

The subperiosteal hemorrhage with a subsequent crater-rim of bone at its outer borders may give the impression of a skull fracture, sometimes raising the question of a depressed skull fracture. This subperiosteal hemorrhage is a benign lesion and does *not* merit skull roentgenograms or other investigative study.

REFERENCE

1. Sterne, L.: The Life and Opinions of Tristram Shandy, Gentleman. Boston, Houghton Mifflin Co., 1965.

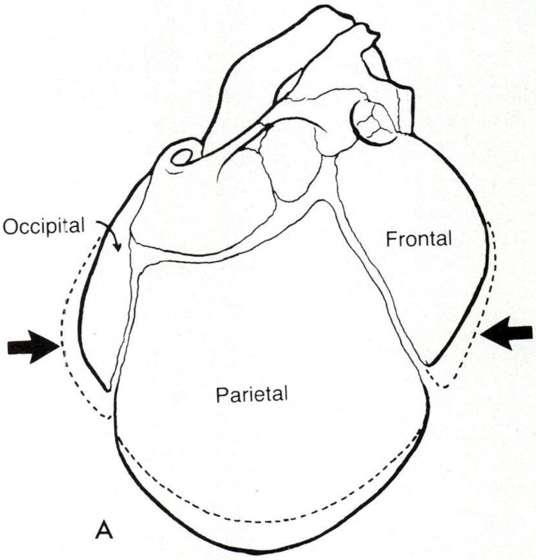

Figure 2–22. Vertex molding. *A,* Nature of forces molding the head during vertex vaginal delivery. The dashed lines show the former contour and the solid lines show the molded contour as the A-P distance is decreased while the head height is increased.

Illustration continued on opposite page

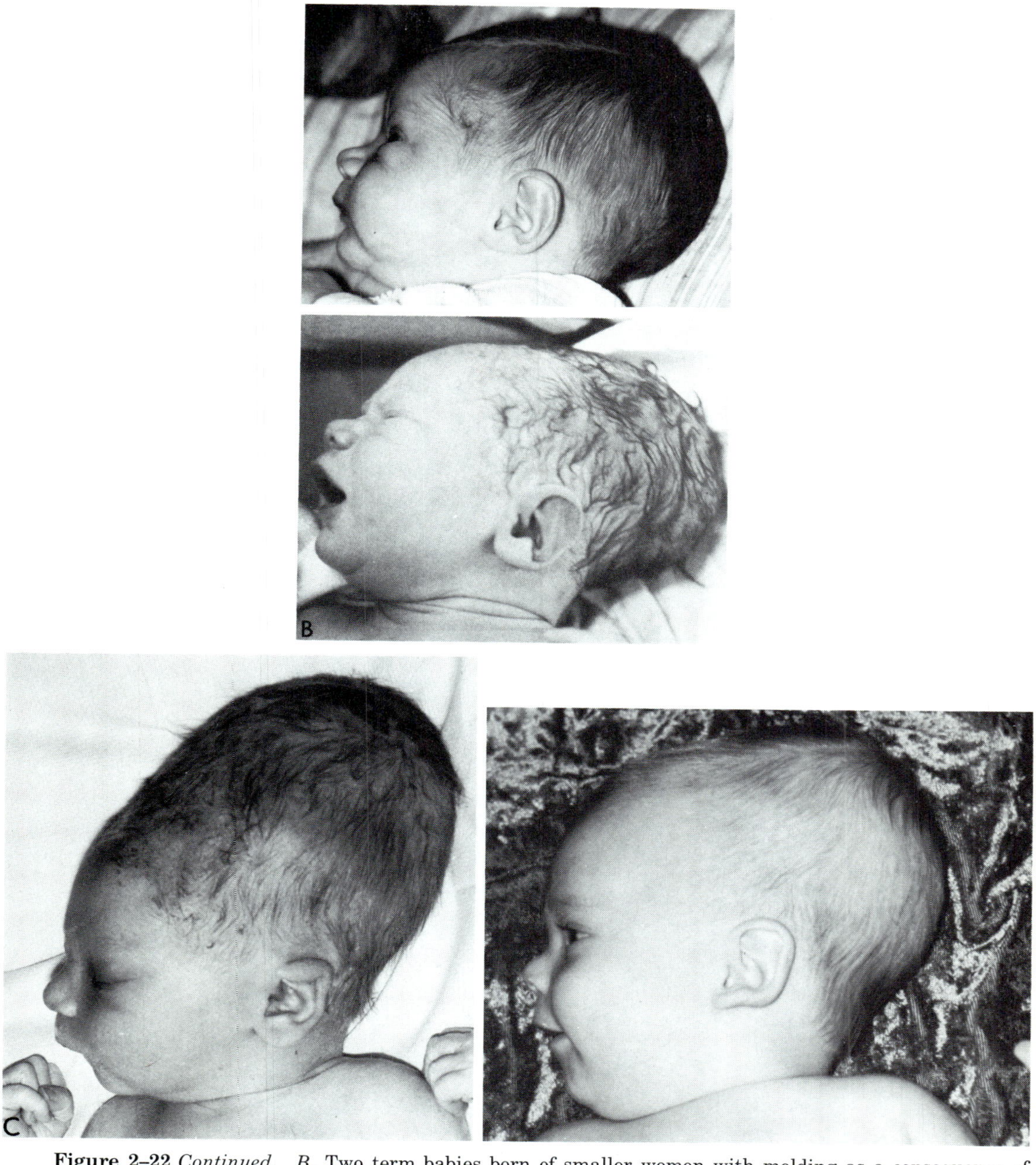

Figure 2–22 *Continued.* *B,* Two term babies born of smaller women with molding as a consequence of cephalopelvic disproportion, *C,* Extreme molding (left), presumably due to a tight cervix that did not fully dilate with the delivery of this large baby. The same baby is shown at 12 weeks of age at the right.

Illustration continued on following page

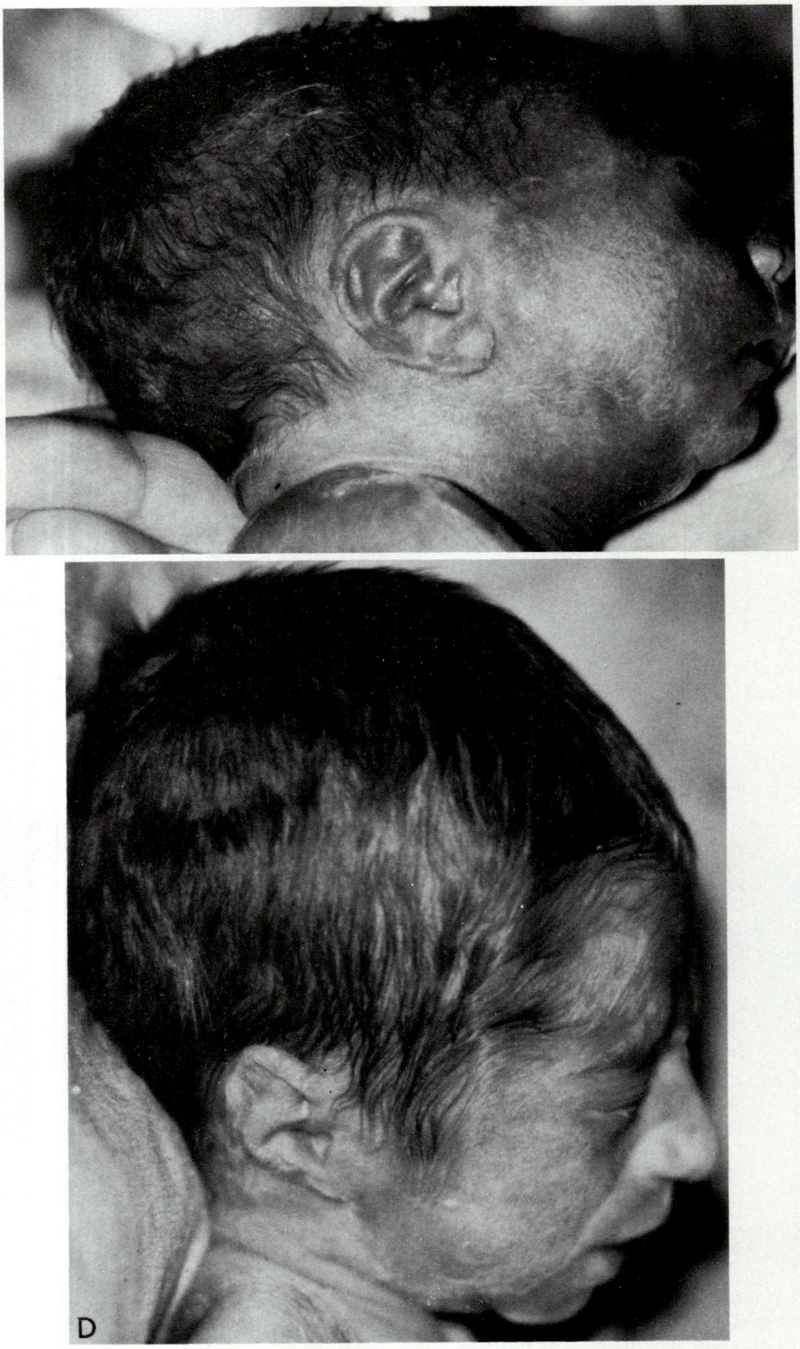

Figure 2–22 *Continued.* *D,* Two prematurely born babies whose more malleable heads are more prone to moderate molding at birth.

13. VERTEX CRANIOTABES

("Soft Head")

GENESIS AND FEATURES. Prolonged forceful pressure on the presenting part, usually the parieto-occipital vertex region, may result in diminished mineralization in the compressed region. This is more likely to occur in a first born, in a large baby, and/or when the maternal pelvic outlet is small. The history often shows that the fetus has dropped (lightening) early and has been in the vertex position in the pelvis for an unusual duration of time. Mild degrees of this compressional craniotabes occur in 2 per cent of newborn babies, and extensive degrees are less common. The parieto-occipital region tends to be soft, and often there is a craniotabes "ping-pong" feel to finger compression. In one extreme instance, the entire top of the head, an area measuring 8 × 10 cm, was involved. The presence of a normally firm bony calvarium along the sides of the calvarium and in the mastoid regions readily differentiates this from the craniotabes that is due to a generalized problem of mineralization, such as in rickets. Within the affected region of the calvarium the sutures and fontanels may feel wider than usual.

Accentuated vertex molding and other features noted in the foregoing section are common features.

The fetus with a vertex craniotabes has often been more constrained than usual in late gestation and may have mild to moderate limitation of full movement in some joints, especially those of the lower limbs.

PROGNOSIS AND COUNSEL. The prognosis is excellent, and the parents may be reassured that the calvarium will mineralize in a normal fashion within one to two months, that there is no risk in handling the "soft head," and that no special precautions are merited.

DIFFERENTIAL DIAGNOSIS. Concern might be generated about problems of mineralization, such as rickets or a skeletal dysplasia. The clinical examination of the whole calvarium will readily resolve such concern. The sides of the calvarium are of normal firmness. Furthermore, there are no problems in skeletal morphogenesis except for the vertex craniotabes. This is not an indication for roentgenograms or for serum calcium phosphorus or alkaline phosphatase studies.

The "soft head" will often convey the impression of open sutures and fontanels, and the question of hydrocephalus or other reasons for increased intracranial pressure may be raised. Such concern may be fostered by the increase in the region of transillumination that may occur when a strong light is held at the soft portion of the calvarium. The head circumference, the head shape, the character of the sutures in the firm portion of the calvarium, and the general clinical status of the infant should resolve these concerns *without* resort to skull roentgenograms or any other studies. If there is concern about a major problem, then close clinical follow-up should resolve the situation with laboratory or roentgenographic studies, since the "soft head" due to compression will normalize postnatally.

REFERENCE

1. Graham, J.M., and Smith, D.W.: Parietal craniotabes in the neonate: Its origin and relevance. J. Pediatr. *95*:114, 1979.

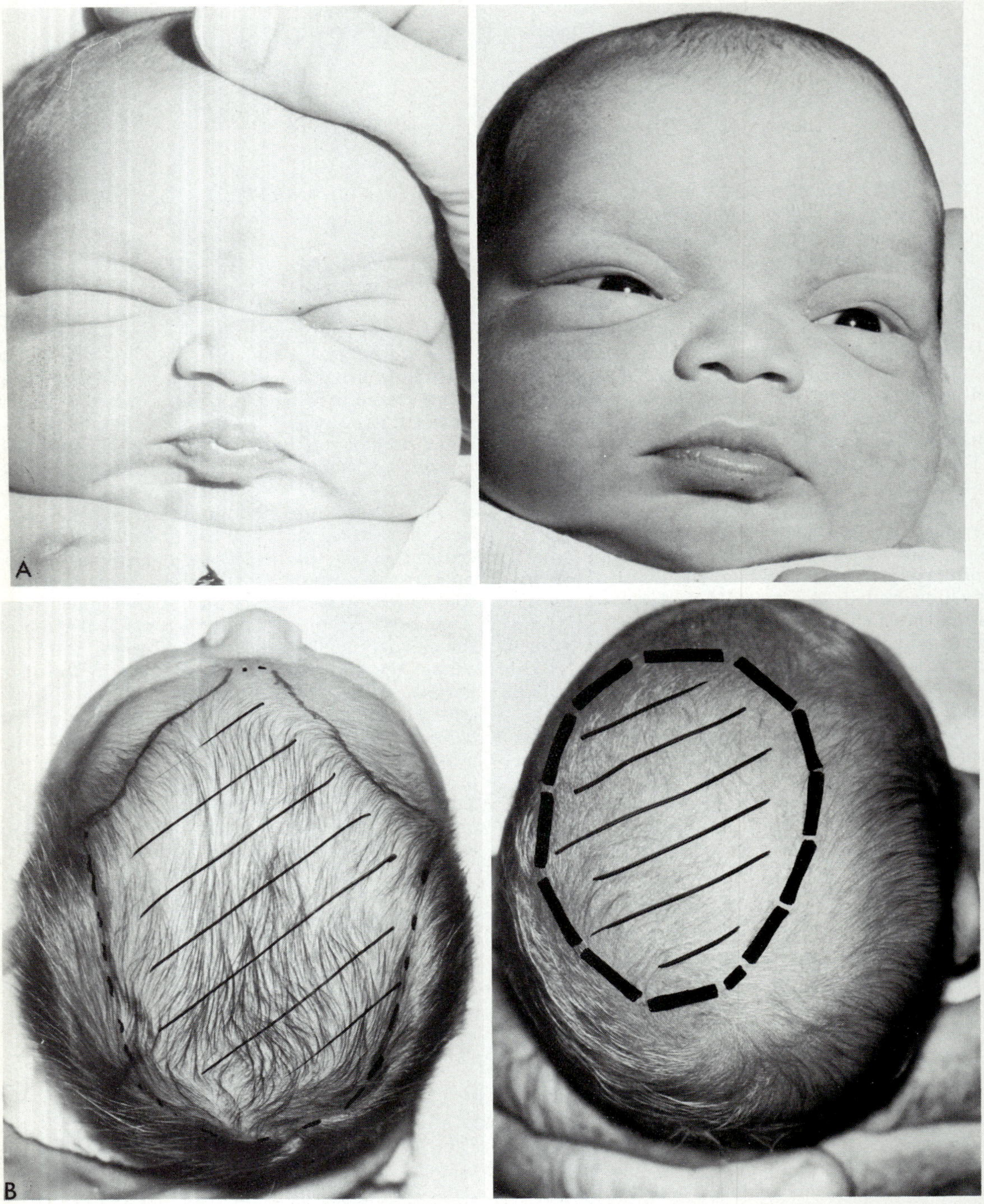

Figure 2–23. Vertex craniotabes, "soft head." *A*, Newborn infant who had been in prolonged vertex position with the head engaged under compression. Relatively forceful pressure by the examiner over the top of the head of the baby (left) did not cause discomfort, this having been the normal situation for the infant in utero. The relative excess of loose facial skin was considered an additional sign of external compression prior to birth. This baby had parietal craniotabes. The mother needs to be reassured that the appearance of the baby will improve immensely! *B*, Areas of soft "ping-pong" craniotabes, shown as hatched areas.

Illustration continued on opposite page

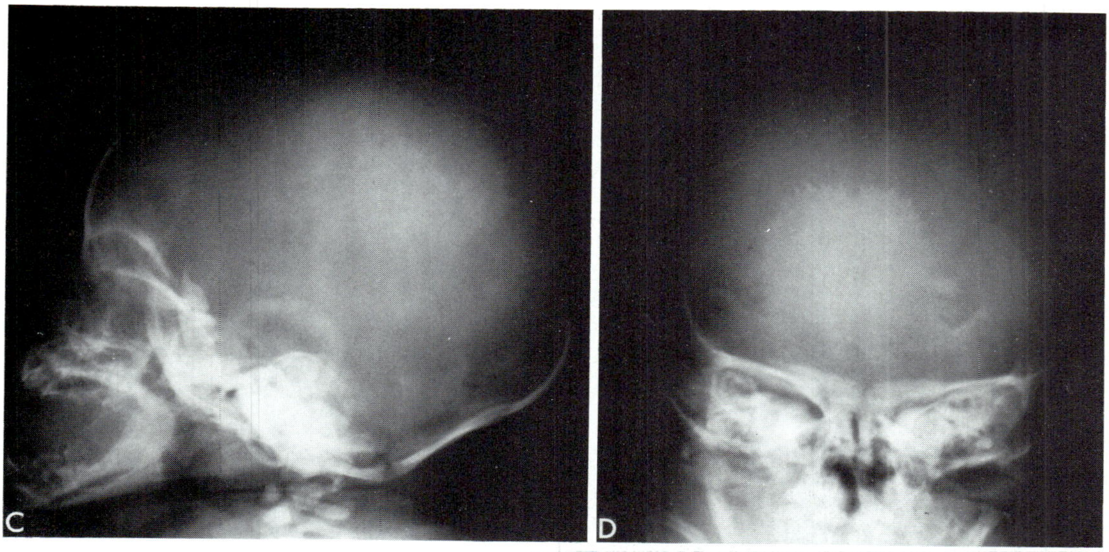

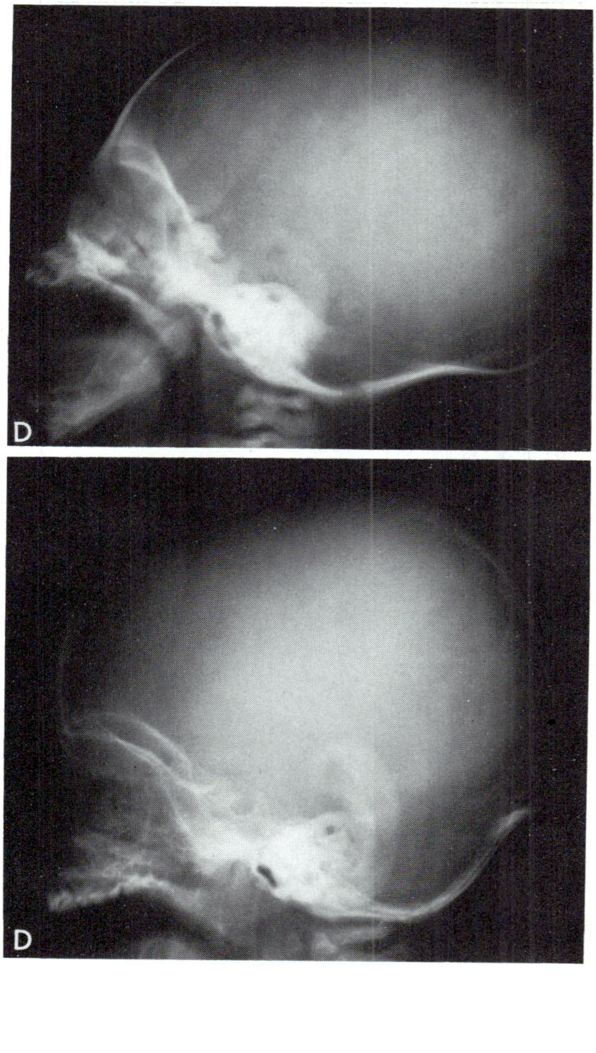

Figure 2–23 *Continued. C,* Diminished mineralization over the vertex in the region of the constraint induced craniotabes. *D,* Molded head with vertex craniotabes at birth (above) and at five weeks of age (below), by which time mineralization is evident in the area of former craniotabes.

14. BREECH PRESENTATION SEQUENCE

GENESIS. Breech position is an important cause of deformation: fully one third of deformations are in babies who have been in the breech position. Since 2 per cent of newly born babies have deformations, this indicates that 0.6 per cent of babies born have one or more deformations because of breech position in utero. Therefore, this is a most important category and will be given extensive coverage.

Some of the causative factors relating to breech position are listed in Table 2–2. It is more common in the primigravida, especially the older woman, than in subsequent pregnancies, presumably because of the difference in the shape of the uterus and in the space for fetal and uterine growth. The spatial situation of twins in utero increases the likelihood of breech presentation, especially for the second in birth order. The prematurely born baby is still moving about in the amniotic fluid and is less likely to have shifted into the vertex birth position. Unless there is oligohydramnios the premature fetus in breech position generally does not have deformations. This is because there has not been sufficient constraint to cause molding. Furthermore, as emphasized, breech presentation is not uncommon as a normal position at this stage of gestation. At 32 weeks of gestation, 25 per cent of fetuses are in the breech presentation position. From this time until birth the majority of fetuses shift into the vertex position. The frequency of breech presentation by term is 3 per cent.[1]

Any situation that causes oligohydramnios, whether it be chronic leakage of amniotic fluid or lack of urine flow into the amniotic space, will restrict movement and greatly increase the chance of the fetus being in the breech presentation position. Alterations of the size and shape of the uterine cavity may also increase the frequency of breech presentation. This may be secondary to a bicornuate uterus or to uterine fibroids, as two examples. The placement of the placenta may be one factor, as emphasized by Kian[3] and summarized in Table 2–3. Placenta previa results in increased breech presentation.

Table 2–2. Frequency of Breech Presentation

All pregnancies	6%
Full term singletons (highest in primigravida women)	3%
Twins	34%
Prematurely born	25%
Oligohydramnios due to chronic leakage	64%
Placenta previa	Increased
Altered shape to uterine cavity, as with bicornuate uterus	Increased
Maternal hypertension	Increased
Malformation of fetus (see Table 2–5)	Increased

Table 2–3. Site of Implantation and Breech Presentation

PER CENT OF ALL PREGNANCIES	SITE OF IMPLANTATION	PER CENT BREECH
66	Cornuo-fundal	4
30	Midwall fundal	20
4	Midwall to low	76

About 70 per cent of fetuses in breech presentation have their legs extended in front of the abdomen.[1] Once "caught" in this position it may be most difficult for the fetus to maneuver out of this particular attitude. Tompkins[4] emphasizes that once the movements of the fetus become limited by extension of the legs in front of the abdomen, the fetus has far less chance of extricating himself or herself from the breech presentation. Dunn has made the analogy to the "folding body press" wrestling hold.[1] Once a wrestler has his opponent in this position with the legs in front of the abdomen there is little the opponent can do to extricate himself or herself.

The breech presentation with the hips flexed and knees extended is termed frank breech, with the hips and knees flexed it is called complete breech, and with hips and knees extended it is referred to as to the footling breech, as depicted in Figure 2–24*C*.

Prolonged breech position in late fetal life will give rise to uterine fundal pressure and molding of the fetal head, which may become retroflexed. This type of constraint results in anterior-posterior elongation of the head with a prominent occipital shelf, the "breech head."[5] The shoulders are often thrust under the auricle and may also distort the mandible. The legs may be caught in front of the fetus, tending to dislocate the hips and occasionally cause genu recurvatum of the knee and often calcaneovalgus position of the feet. In the complete breech position with the legs flexed across the abdomen, the feet are liable to be compressed into an equinovarus position. The genital region, as the presenting part, may be molded and edematous.

Dunn[1] noted that 32 per cent of all deformations in the newly born baby related to breech presentation in utero. In his series of more than 6000 babies, 100 per cent of genu recurvatum cases related to breech, as did 50 per cent of hip dislocation cases, 42 per cent of postural scoliosis cases, and 20 to 25 per cent each for cases of mandibular asymmetry, torticollis, and talipes equinovarus. This is illustrated in Figure 2–24*A*.

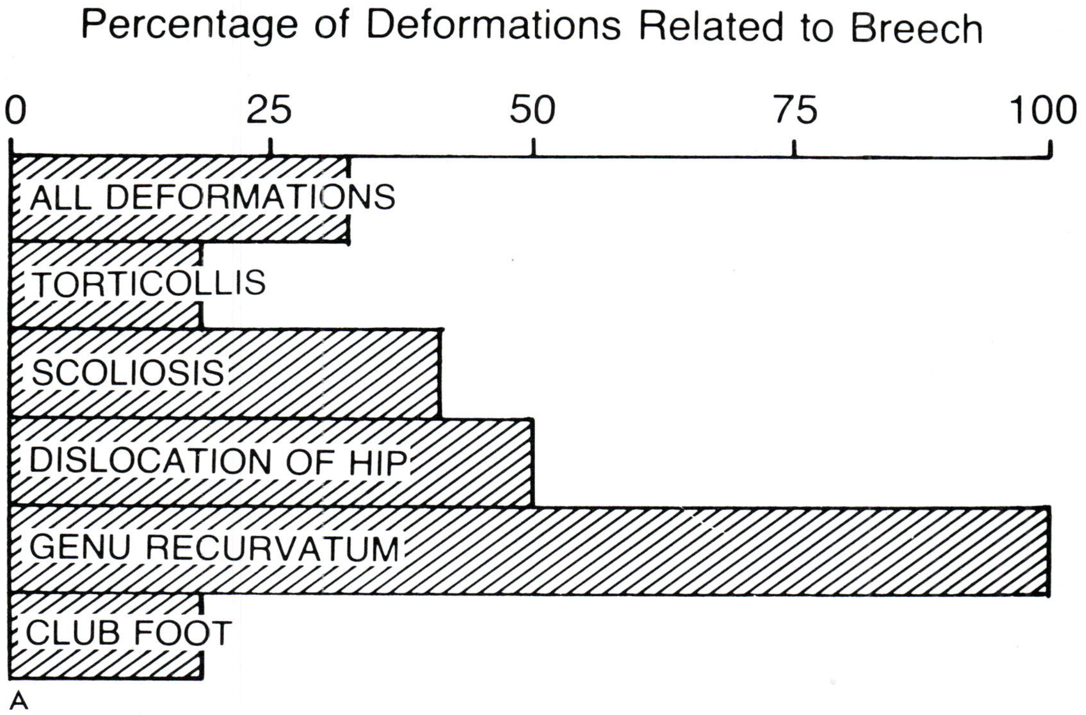

Figure 2–24. Breech presentation deformation sequence. *A*, The percentage of breech presentations in association with particular deformations in the study of Dunn on some 6000 newborn infants. (From Dunn, P. M.: 5th European Congress of Perinatology, Uppsala, Sweden, p. 76, 1976.)

Illustration continued on page 70

FEATURES

Craniofacial. The head is often elongated toward a scaphocephalic form, often with a prominent occipital shelf. There may be redundant folds of skin in the posterior neck, the presumed result of compression due to retroflexion of the head. The lambdoid sutures may be overlapping and/or ridged because of the fetal head constraint. The lower auricle may be forced upward into the location where the shoulder has been, and there may be a "hollow" appearance at the manubrial region of the mandible. The shoulder compression is often asymmetrical, and hence there may be asymmetry of the mandible with an "upward tilt" on the more compressed side. Torticollis may occur secondary to traumatic tearing of the sternocleidomastoid muscle during vaginal delivery.

Limbs. All gradations of hip dislocation may occur in breech presentation and are considered to be the consequence of the constrained position in utero which forces the hip from its usual socket. The legs have generally been hyperflexed in front of the fetus, and this is often the "position of comfort" in the early neonatal period. As one consequence it may be difficult to fully extend and abduct the hips into the position that is usually utilized for detecting dislocation of the hips. There also may be some limitation in the full movement at the knees. This is the most common cause of genu recurvatum. The extended leg position may lead to calcaneovalgus foot deformity, while the flexed leg position more commonly leads to an equinovarus foot deformity.

Genitalia. The buttocks and genitalia tend to be the leading parts at delivery and may show edema and/or bruising. Secondary hydrocele of the testicle is frequent.

COMPLICATIONS OF BREECH BESIDES DEFORMATIONS. It is important to emphasize some of the complications that can ensue in the vaginal delivery of a baby in breech presentation. The risk of vaginal delivery must be weighed in each case against the risk of cesarean section. As more cesarean sections are being done for breech presentation, especially in the primigravida, the frequency of serious complications has fallen. Perinatal mortality was 13 per cent for breech presentation, much of which was accounted for by prematurely born infants, twins, and babies with malformations.[2] It is important to appreciate that the premature baby is more likely to be in the breech position in early gestation. However, it is also important to realize that the breech position *itself* is frequently associated with premature labor. The overall frequency of breech presentation in premature deliveries from 28 to 36 weeks' gestation is 24 per cent. For the term singleton breech without malformation the perinatal mortality is 1 per cent.[2] The breech fetus is more likely to have its head become entrapped during the second stage of labor, which tends to increase the frequency of tentorial tears and intracranial bleeding, asphyxia (five to six times greater risk), and trauma relating to the attempt to "pull" the infant out.[2] Serious consequences include trauma to the spinal cord, to the brachial plexus (Erb's or Klumpke's paresis), and/or compression of the vertebral artery with cerebral ischemia. The gravest concern is with vaginal delivery of the breech fetus who has a hyperextended head, which occurs in at least 5 per cent of breech fetuses. Of those who failed to revert to nonextended head position and were delivered by the vaginal route, 21 per cent had upper spinal cord transection.[6] The acute symptoms of such transection are usually respiratory problems, a weak cry, poor muscle tone, poor feeding, and often death. The survivors are usually severely debilitated with spastic quadriplegia. Lesser degrees of cord damage at C5 to C6 may produce hand and forearm weakness with flexor weakness and wristdrop. Less commonly, the damage is at the C8 to T1 cord level, yielding extensor weakness with the fingers and hands ventriflexed. About 50 per cent of infants with so-called Erb's and Klumpke's pareses recover, usually by three to five months of age. Compression of the vertebral artery may occur, yielding secondary problems in the medullary area of the brain. A significant proportion of cerebral palsy of the past may relate to problems engendered by breech presentation with vaginal delivery. The late Dr. Nicholson Eastman of Johns Hopkins Hospital estimated that 24 per cent of cerebral palsy was on this basis.

Fractures of the femur, humerus, and clavicle are more common, as is bruising with secondary hyperbilirubinemia.[2] Tears of muscles may occur, and 20 per cent of instances of torticollis are in babies who were in breech presentation.

Another complication that may be secondary to breech vaginal delivery trauma is severance of the pituitary stalk with consequent hypopituitarism.[7] Vaginal breech delivery appears to be one of the most common causes of hypopituitarism, realizing that hypopituitarism is relatively rare.

MANAGEMENT, PROGNOSIS, AND COUNSEL. In the prevention and management of breech presentation, three factors must be considered. First is prevention of the deformities and complications of vaginal delivery by moving the fetus into the vertex position long before the time of delivery by a method referred to as external cephalic version. Second is avoidance of the complications that relate to vaginal delivery of the breech fetus by accomplishing the delivery by cesarean section. Third is the management of any deformations and complications after delivery of the breech fetus.

External Cephalic Version. External cephalic version, the external manipulation of the fetus from the breech or transverse position into the vertex position, is a controversial procedure that is seldom taught as a part of obstetrics training today.[8] The major concern about the procedure is the potential risk to the fetus and mother versus the value of this measure. The procedural risk figures vary from zero to several per cent fetal mortality from such problems as early separation of the placenta, cord compression or prolapse, early rupture of membranes, and premature delivery.[8-10] In one study the overall complication rate was 4.4 per cent, which included fetal death in 0.9 per cent, premature labor in 1.2 per cent, and antepartum hemorrhage in 1.3 per cent. In addition, the attempt to accomplish external version is not always successful and the fetus may revert back into the breech position before birth. Considering the other side of the question, successful external version limits the need for cesarean section and negates the risk of the deformities and complications involved in the vaginal delivery of a fetus in breech position. The success rate with external version varies from about 30 to 98 per cent. The latter figure was obtained by Dr. Brooks Ranney of South Dakota, who accomplished 1240 external cephalic versions without a recognized complication for either the fetus or the pregnant woman.[11] Nearly two thirds of these fetuses reverted to an abnormal presentation and required repeat version. His recommendations include performing the version before 34 weeks of gestation. The mean age of version in his practice was 31 weeks. If one waits until after 34 to 35 weeks the size of the fetus in relation to the amount of amniotic fluid is such that successful and safe version is difficult. A second recommendation is that the maneuver be gentle. Neither analgesia nor anesthesia should be utilized. If gentle maneuvering does not work, the procedure should be stopped and tried again in a few days. External version should not be attempted if there are twins, if there is serious oligohydramnios, if the membranes have ruptured, if there is obvious placenta previa, or if the woman has diabetes mellitus, hypertension, or is Rh sensitized.

Utilizing external cephalic version Dr. Ranney[11] reduced the frequency of breech presentation at birth from 4 per cent to 1 per cent and the frequency of prematurity related to breech or transverse presentation from 18 per cent to 3 per cent. The frequency of need for cesarean section was markedly reduced and the perinatal mortality was reduced. It must be appreciated that these are the best results ever reported and that other observers have not had as great success with this maneuver. Though other physicians[12] have had results somewhat similar to those of Ranney, it is

Table 2-4. Factors Favoring Cesarean Section[1, 5, 12-14] Delivery of the Fetus in Breech Presentation

1. Scaphocephalic "breech head"
2. Hyperextended head
3. Contracted pelvis
4. Large baby, over 4.0 kg
5. Small baby, under 2.5 kg
6. Placenta previa
7. Maternal hypertension
8. Uterine dysfunction
9. Primigravida, especially if 35 years or older
10. Footling breech presentation
11. Previous pregnancy wastage

important to appreciate that most physicians are not experienced in performing the maneuver.

Cesarean Section. Given a fetus in breech presentation, the second line of prevention is to strive to forestall the potential complications of vaginal delivery by accomplishing a cesarean section when indicated.[1, 13-15] Table 2–4 lists some of the indications for a cesarean delivery. As the concern for the complications of vaginal delivery of the breech fetus have increased in recent years, so also has the frequency of cesarean section for breech presentation. As previously mentioned, prolonged breech in late fetal life tends to lead to a scaphocephalic "breech head," a deformity that enhances the risk of vaginal delivery. Sonography or roentgenography can be utilized to ascertain the extent of molding of the calvarium toward this elongated "breech head." Its recognition may be used as an additional clue toward utilization of cesarean section rather than vaginal delivery. The scaphocephaly with prominent occipital shelf may create a serious problem in bringing the aftercoming head through the cervical opening. Such a head is more likely to become stuck during the second stage of labor. Attempts at extraction from below will enhance the risk of neurological damage, such as brachial plexus palsy, cord tears, and/or temporary vertebral artery occlusion with potentially serious consequences.

MANAGEMENT OF DEFORMATIONS AND COMPLICATIONS. After birth the head shape as well as mandibular form gradually returns to normal with no management being indicated.

If the hips are dislocated, a more rigorous management is indicated.

The hydrocele of the testis is a benign lesion that rarely merits therapy.

Tears of muscles may occur and 20 per cent of instances of torticollis are in babies who were in breech position.

DIFFERENTIAL DIAGNOSIS. The most important question about the infant with the breech deformation complex is did an otherwise normal infant become caught in the breech presentation, in which instance the prognosis, without birth complications, is usually excellent, or was the infant in the breech presentation *because* of a fetal problem? If the infant is in the latter category, the prognosis relates predominantly to the basic diagnosis, with the addition of the secondary deformities due to breech presentation and/or the disruptive complications that may occur with vaginal delivery. The overall frequency of breech presentation in newborn babies with malformation problems is 23 per cent,[2] about eight times the general frequency. Such patients account for a sizeable proportion of the excess mortality of babies born in breech position. Certain categories of malformation problems are notorious for failing to accommodate to a vertex position. The cause may be a structural defect, a neuromuscular defect, a renal defect resulting in oligohydramnios, or a problem of crowding. Table 2–5 lists some of the defects in which breech is a frequent consequence.

The elongated scaphocephalic head may also be due to a sagittal craniostenosis problem. Usually palpation of the normally mobile sagittal suture is all that is required. Any doubt that might exist may generally be resolved by the follow-up, which

Table 2–5. Malformation Disorders That Predispose to Breech Presentation[1, 5]

DISORDER	BREECH FREQUENCY	EXPLANATION
Lower limb deficiency	60%	Lack of leg thrust
Meningomyelocele in general	48%	Lack of leg thrust
Meningomyelocele with leg paralysis	93%	Lack of leg thrust
Anencephaly	excess	Neurological deficiency
Prader-Willi syndrome	50%	Neurological deficiency
Smith-Lemli-Opitz syndrome	40%	Neurological deficiency
Renal agenesis	50%	Oligohydramnios with limited mobility
Severe polycystic kidneys	excess	Oligohydramnios with limited mobility
Urethral obstruction	excess	Oligohydramnios with limited mobility
Bicornuate uterus	excess	Crowding with limited mobility

shows progressive improvement toward normal form for the molded "breech head." Roentgenograms are generally not indicated.

The shape of the head may yield a spuriously high occipitofrontal head circumference, raising concern about hydrocephalus or macrocephaly. Generally this question can be readily resolved by simple examination of the head and sutures without further studies.

Dislocation of the hip may be engendered by a number of causes. When there is a basic problem in connective tissue that enhances the likelihood of mechanical dislocation, joints other than the hip are usually hypermobile. In the usual breech presentation patient who has dislocation of the hips the joints are generally *less* mobile than usual, as a result of prolonged deficit in full range of movement.

Finally, the multiple consequences of prolonged breech presentation may be mistakenly interpreted as a multiple malformation disorder.

REFERENCES

1. Dunn, P.M.: Maternal and fetal aetiological factors. 5th European Congress of Perinatal Medicine, Uppsala, Sweden, 1976, p. 76.
2. Dunn, P.M.: Breech delivery: Perinatal morbidity and mortality. 5th European Congress of Perinatal Medicine, Uppsala, Sweden, 1976, p. 54.
3. Kian, L.S.: The role of the placental site in the etiology of breech presentation. J. Obstet. Gynaecol. Brit. Cwlth. *70*:795, 1963.
4. Tompkins, P.: An inquiry into the causes of breech presentation. Am. J. Obstet. Gynecol. *51*:595, 1946.
5. Haberkern, C., Smith, D.W., and Jones, K.L.: The "breech head" and its relevance. Am. J. Dis. Child. *133*:154, 1979.
6. Cimmino, C.V., and Southworth, L.E.: Persistent hyperextension of the neck in breech and transverse lie: Indication for cesarean section. Am. J. Roentgenol. *125*:447, 1975.
7. Rona, R.J., and Tanner, J.M.: Aetiology of idiopathic growth hormone deficiency in England and Wales. Arch. Dis. Child. *52*:197, 1977.
8. Bradley-Watson, P.J.: The decreasing value of external cephalic version in modern obstetric practice. Am. J. Obstet. Gynecol. *123*:237, 1975.
9. Friedlander, D.: External cephalic version in the management of breech presentation. A report of 706 patients treated by this method. Am. J. Obstet. Gynecol. *95*:906, 1966.
10. Hibbard, L.T., and Schumann, W.R.: Prophylactic cephalic version in an obstetric practice. Am. J. Obstet. Gynecol. *116*:511, 1973.
11. Ranney, B.: The gentle art of external cephalic version. Am. J. Obstet. Gynecol. *116*:239, 1973.
12. Bock, J.E.: The influence of prophylactic external cephalic version on the incidence of breech delivery. Acta Obstet. Gynec. Scand. *48*:215, 1969.
13. Butler, N.R., and Bonham, D.G.: Perinatal mortality. The first report of the 1958 Perinatal Mortality Survey. London, E & S Livingstone, Ltd., 1963.
14. Hall, J.E., Kohl, S.G., O'Brien, F., and Ginsberg, M.: Breech presentation and perinatal mortality. A study of 6,044 cases. Am. J. Obstet. Gynecol. *91*:665, 1965.
15. Rovinsky, J.J., Miller, J.A., and Kaplan, S.: Management of breech presentation at term. Am. J. Obstet. Gynecol. *115*:497,1973.

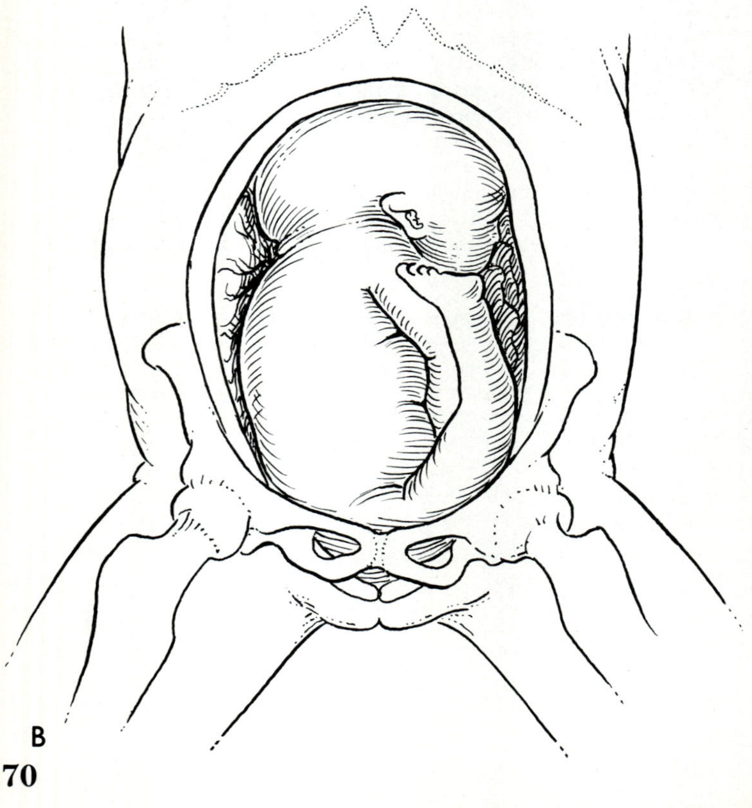

Figure 2–24 *Continued. B,* Frank breech presentation in utero in a term infant. (Adapted from in-utero roentgenograms and postnatal photos of Dunn, P. M.: Growth retardation of infants with congenital postural deformities. Acta Med. Auxol. 7:63, 1975.)

Illustration continued on opposite page

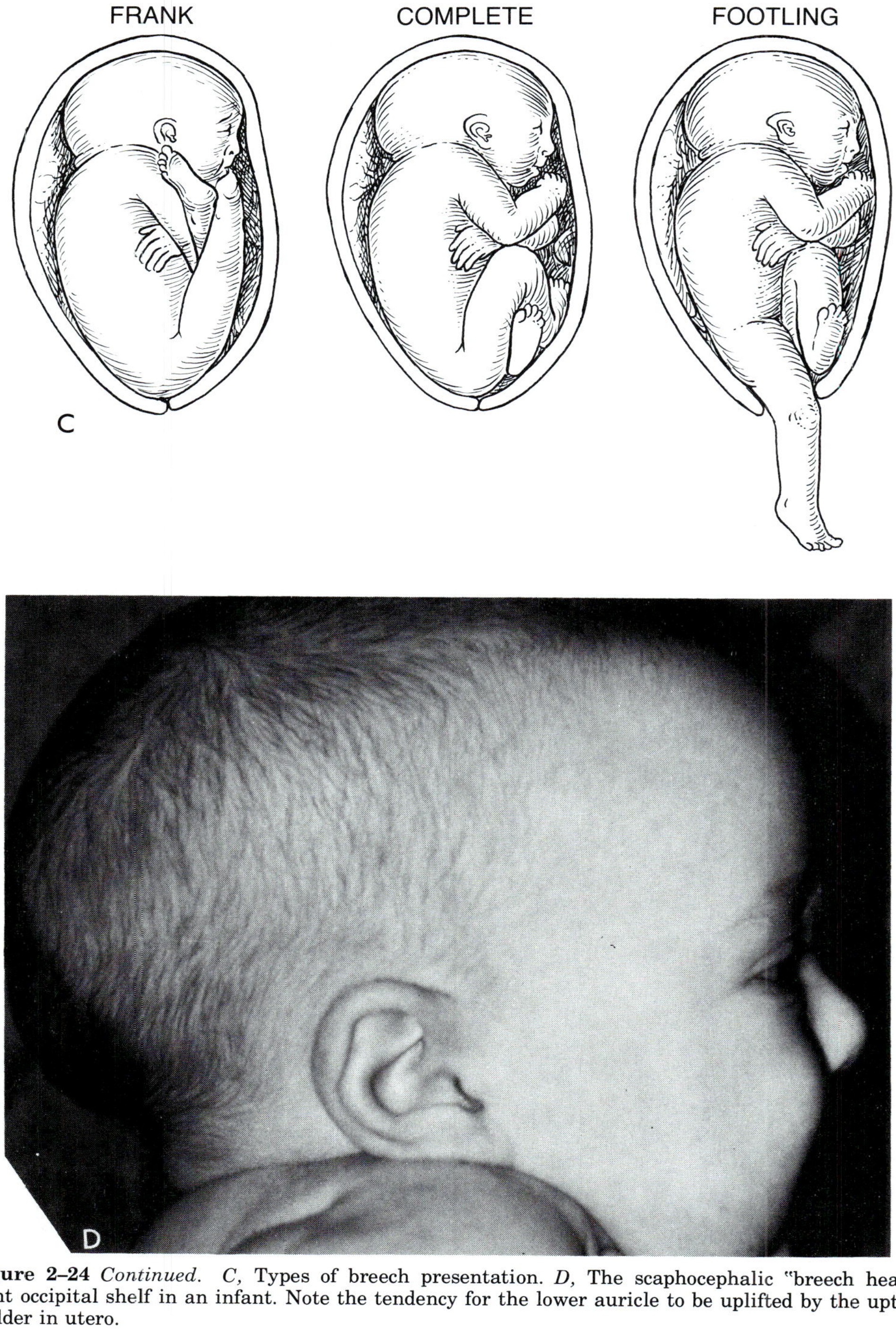

Figure 2–24 *Continued.* *C,* Types of breech presentation. *D,* The scaphocephalic "breech head" with prominent occipital shelf in an infant. Note the tendency for the lower auricle to be uplifted by the upthrust of the shoulder in utero.

Illustration continued on following page

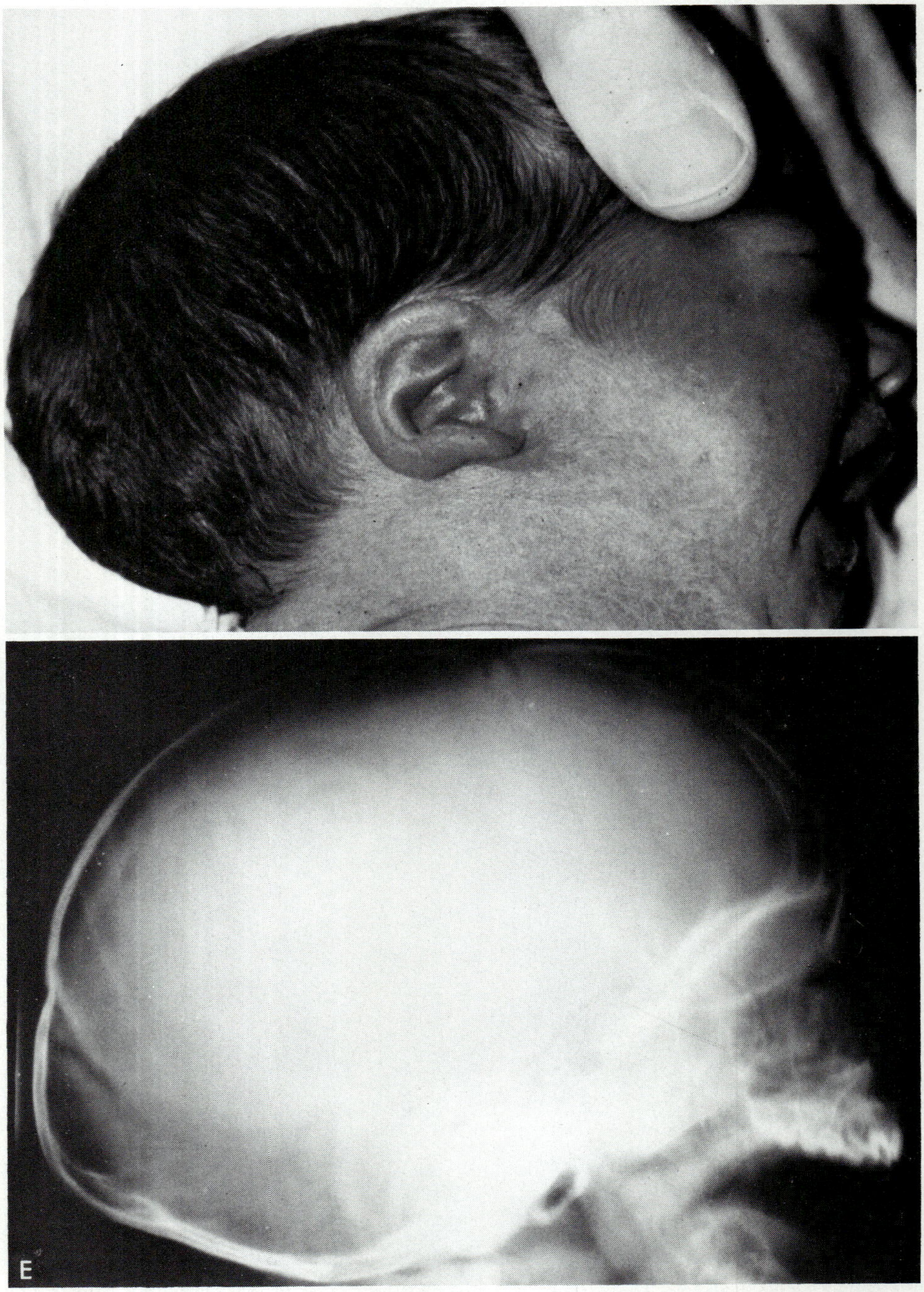

Figure 2–24 *Continued.* *E,* "Breech" head. Note the prominent occipital shelf which is evident by roentgenography.

Illustration continued on opposite page

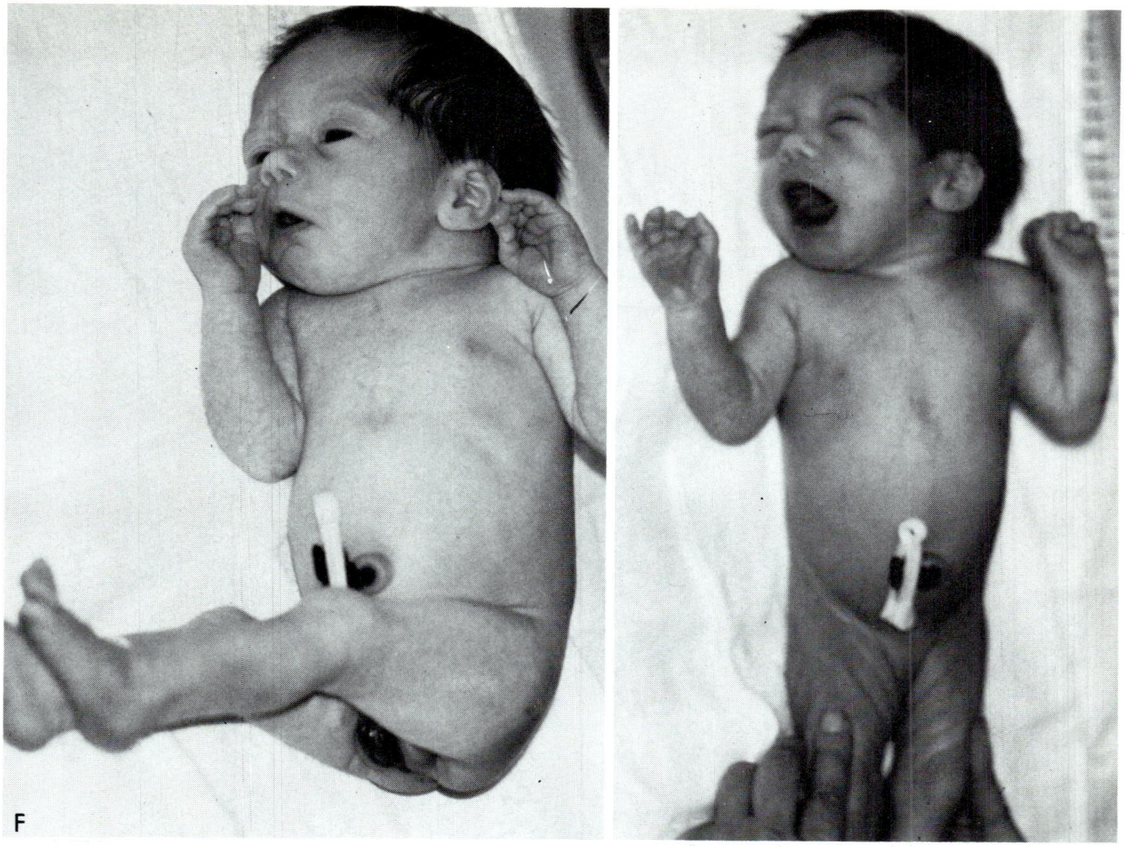

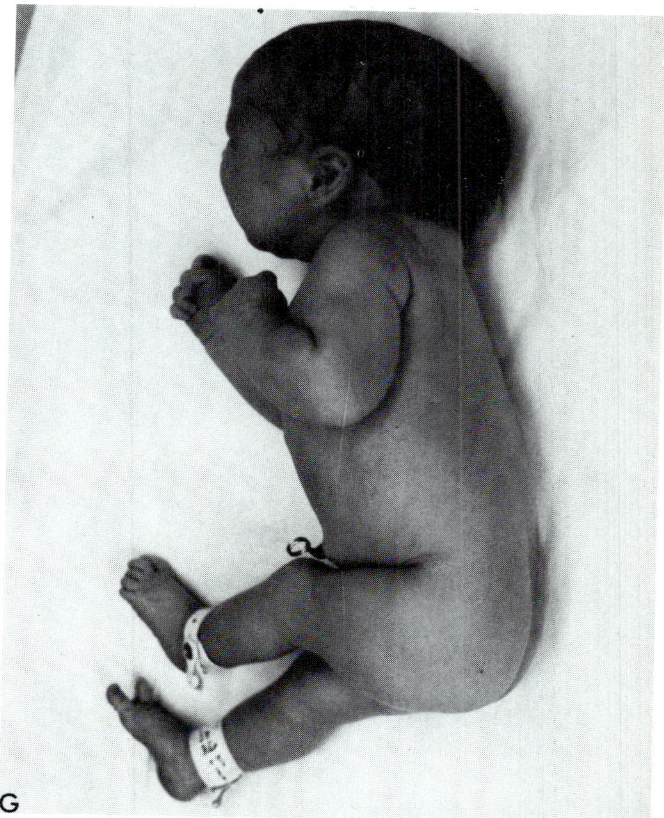

Figure 2–24 *Continued. F,* Newborn baby who had been in the breech presentation in utero showing flexed hips and extended knees in the "position of comfort" and great discomfort when the thighs are extended. *G,* Extended knees and flexed thighs in a baby who had been in prolonged breech presentation and had bilaterally dislocated hips. Note the "breech head."
Illustration continued on following page

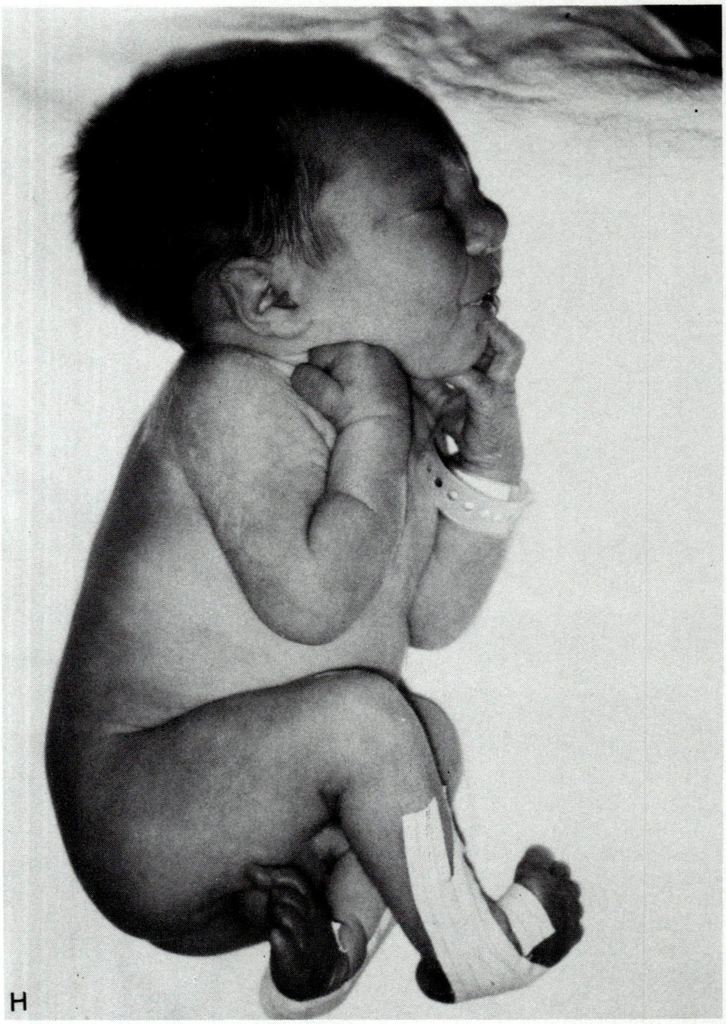

Figure 2–24 *Continued.* *H,* Infant who had been in frank breech presentation with flexed thighs and flexed lower legs. The equinovarus foot deformations, being treated by taping, are considered secondary to the complete breech presentation. Note the "breech head."

Illustration continued on opposite page

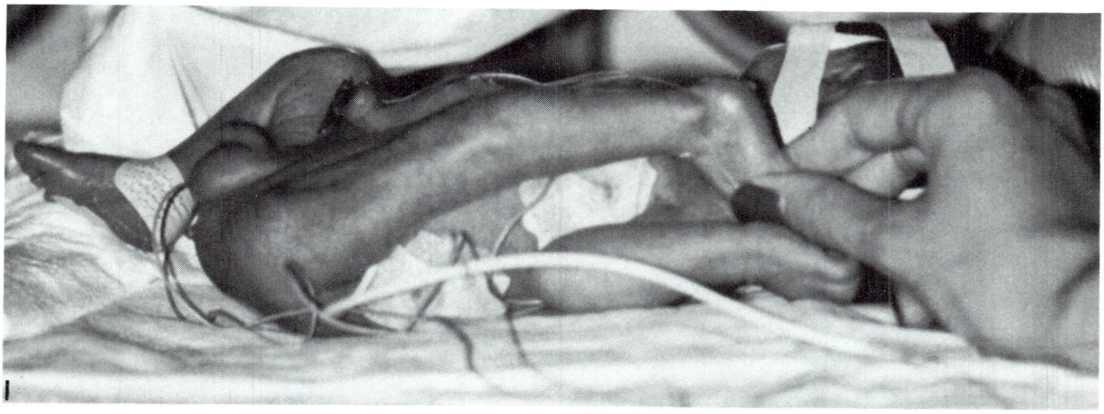

I

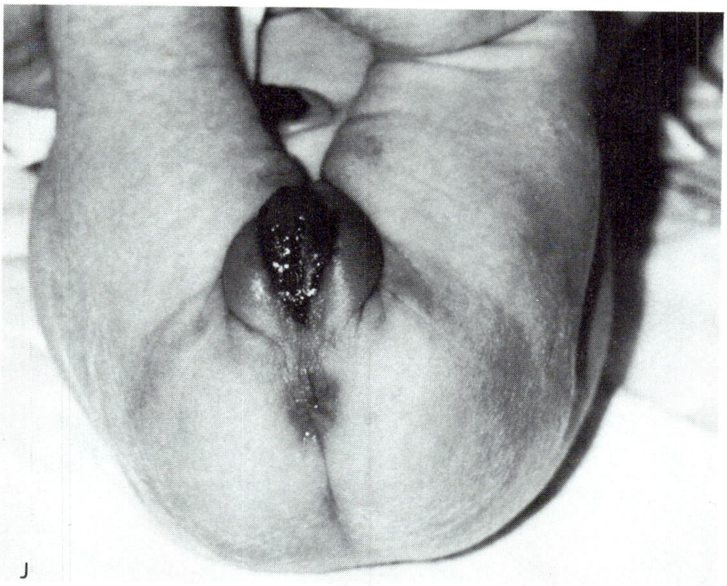

J

Figure 2–24 *Continued.* *I,* Prematurely born infant who had been in frank breech presentation shows genu recurvatum as a consequence. *J,* The edematous swelling of the labia majora and hemorrhagic edematous swelling of the labia minora and external vagina are secondary to prolonged constraint of this presenting part in the frank presentation. Look carefully for the ringlike zone around the buttocks and including the genitalia, which apparently represent the site of cervix indentation on the presenting part.

15. TRANSVERSE PRESENTATION

COMMENT. Transverse lie is fortunately rare, occurring once in about every 300 to 600 deliveries. It is more common in multiparous women. Most of the data regarding breech position are also applicable to transverse presentation. Hence only a few comments will be set forth.

GENESIS AND FEATURES. The lateral constraint may flatten the face, limit mandibular growth, cause a retroflexed head, and lead to scoliosis as well as other deformations.

MANAGEMENT. Similar to breech position. Again, external cephalic version, a controversial procedure, merits consideration. However, it must be remembered that two common causes of transverse presentation, namely inlet contraction and placenta previa, would normally preclude vaginal delivery. Unresolved transverse presentation is usually an indication for cesarean section delivery.

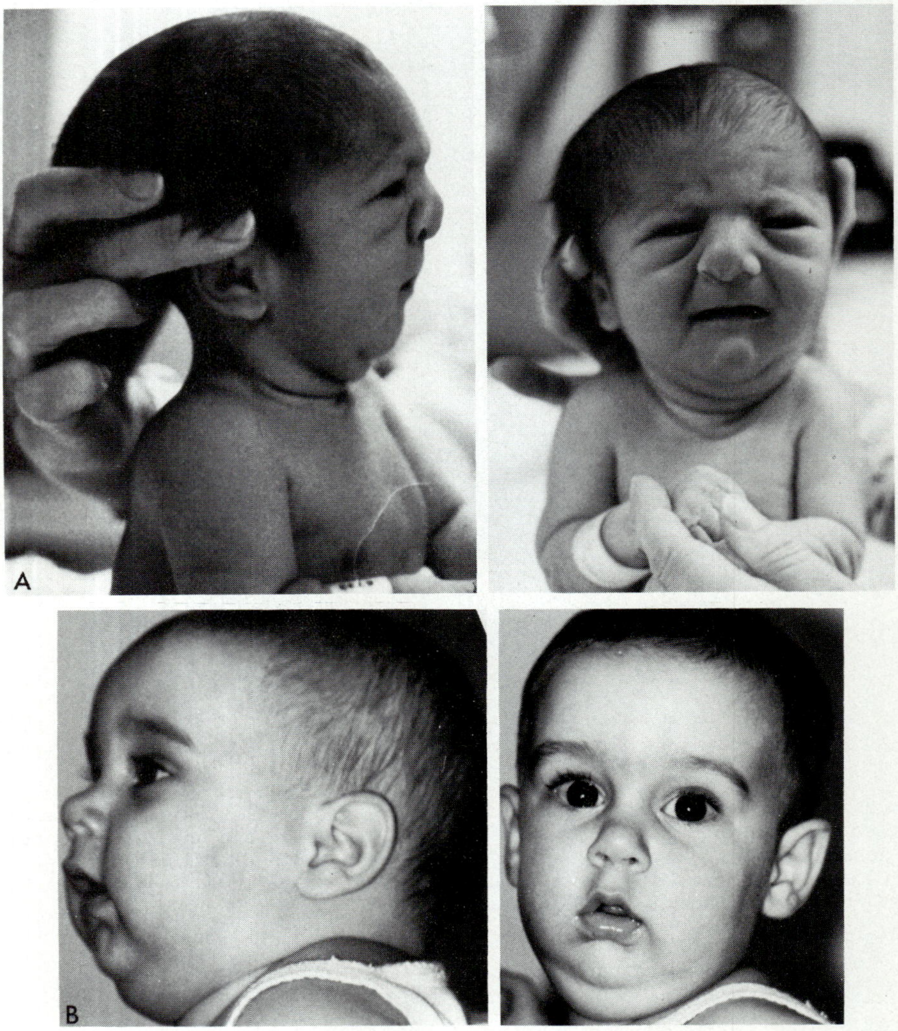

Figure 2–25. *A*, Flattening of the face with redundant "compression" skin in facies plus equinivarus foot deformities in an infant who had been in prolonged transverse presentation, apparently with the head retroflexed and the face forced against the wall of the uterus. The mother could be reassured that the infant will appear progressively better and return to normal form. (Courtesy of Dr. John Carey, from University of California Medical School, San Francisco.) *B,* Same infant at several months of age showing spontaneous resolution toward normal form.

Illustration continued on opposite page

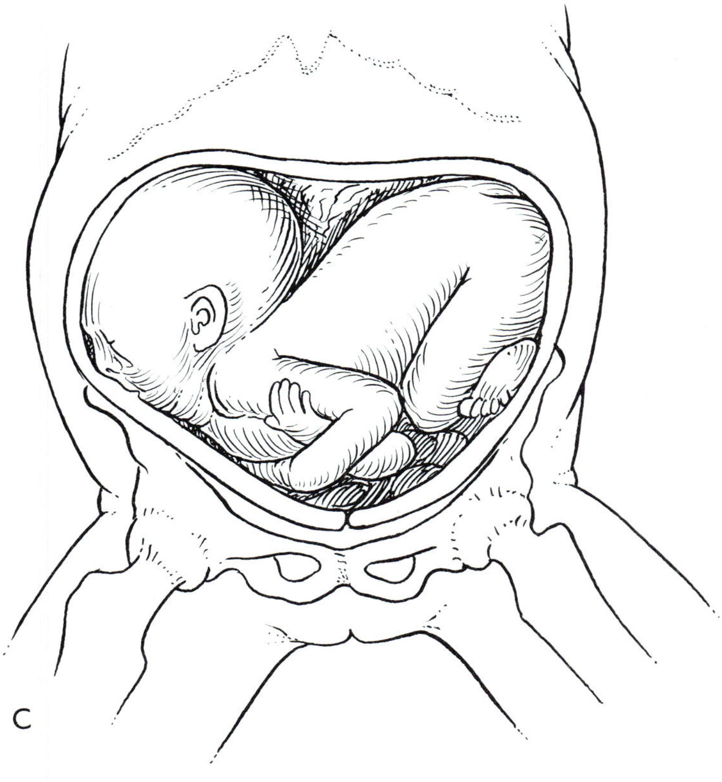

C

Figure 2–25 *Continued.* *C,* Transverse presentation.

16. FACE AND BROW PRESENTATION DEFORMATION

GENESIS. In this presentation the face is the compressed presenting part, usually with extension of the head. Face presentation occurs about once in 500 births, and persistent brow presentation is even less common.

FEATURES

Face Presentation. The growth of the mandible and nose may be restrained. The neck is often retroflexed, the position of comfort for the baby after birth. As a consequence of compression of the chin region and the retroflexion and stretching of the skin of the anterior neck there tend to be redundant folds of skin in the anterior upper neck.

Brow Presentation. The brow is unusually prominent, whereas the midface is less prominent than usual.

Face and brow presentation carry an increased risk of prematurity and of difficult labor. Compression of the neck against the pubic ramus during delivery can cause fracture of the trachea or the larynx. Cesarean section merits consideration, especially if the fetus is large or if the mother has a relatively small pelvis. Only anterior positions can be delivered vaginally because of the inability of the fetal neck to further extend in the posterior position.

MANAGEMENT AND PROGNOSIS. Postnatally there tends to be catch-up of the restrained facial growth toward normal. The head gradually resumes a more normal posture and the infant "grows into" the redundant skin that may be present on the anterior neck (face presentation). The parents need to be reassured that the infant is normal. There is generally no significant recurrent risk.

DIFFERENTIAL DIAGNOSIS

Face Presentation. The appearance of the face at birth may raise the question of a malformation problem such as Treacher-Collins syndrome or other craniofacial dysostosis. The malformation of the auricle and lower lid of Treacher-Collins syndrome tends to distinguish the two types of disorder, as does a history of face presentation and the progressive postnatal improvement with the face presentation deformation sequence.

Brow Presentation. The appearance of the facies may suggest a craniofacial dysostosis problem such as Crouzon syndrome.

A major proportion of face presentation cases are anencephalic infants. Ninety per cent of deaths of babies born in face or brow presentation are infants with major malformation(s).

REFERENCES

1. von Reuss, A.R.: The Diseases of the Newborn. New York, William Wood and Co., 1921.
2. Butler, N.R., and Bonham, D.G.: Perinatal Mortality. The First Report of the 1958 British Perinatal Mortality Survey. London, E & S Livingstone Ltd., 1963.
3. Greenhill, J.P., and Friedman, E.A.: Biological Principles and Modern Practice of Obstetrics. Philadelphia, W. B. Saunders Co., 1974.

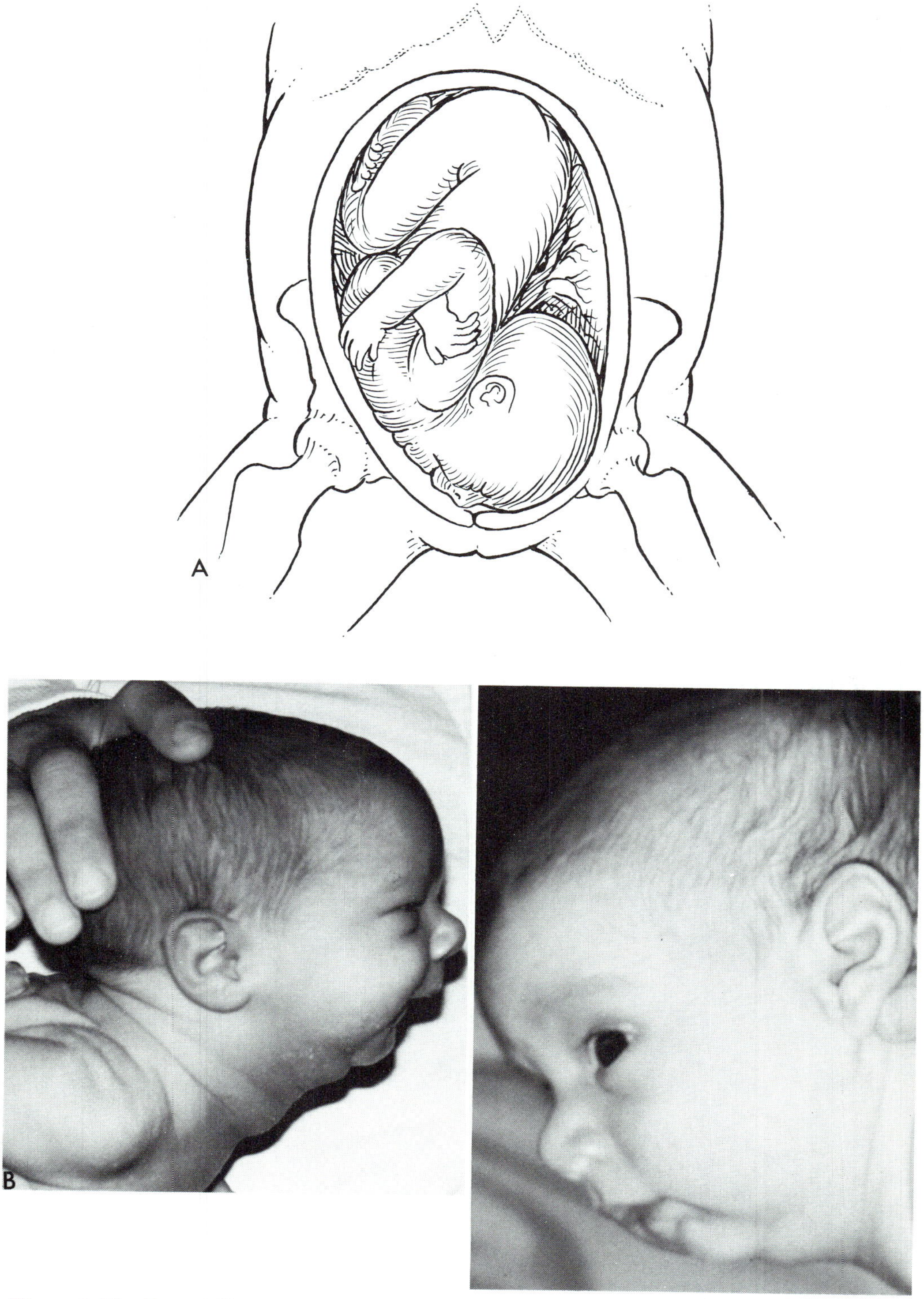

Figure 2–26. Face and brow presentation deformation. *A,* Face presentation. *B,* Newborn infant of a small primigravida mother. The infant was in face presentation for at least the last two months of gestation, producing the extended head, the restriction of nasal and mandibular growth, and the compressive overgrowth of skin in the anterior neck. By six weeks of age, the catch-up growth of the nose and mandible are evident and the head is coming into a more normal alignment.

Illustration continued on following page

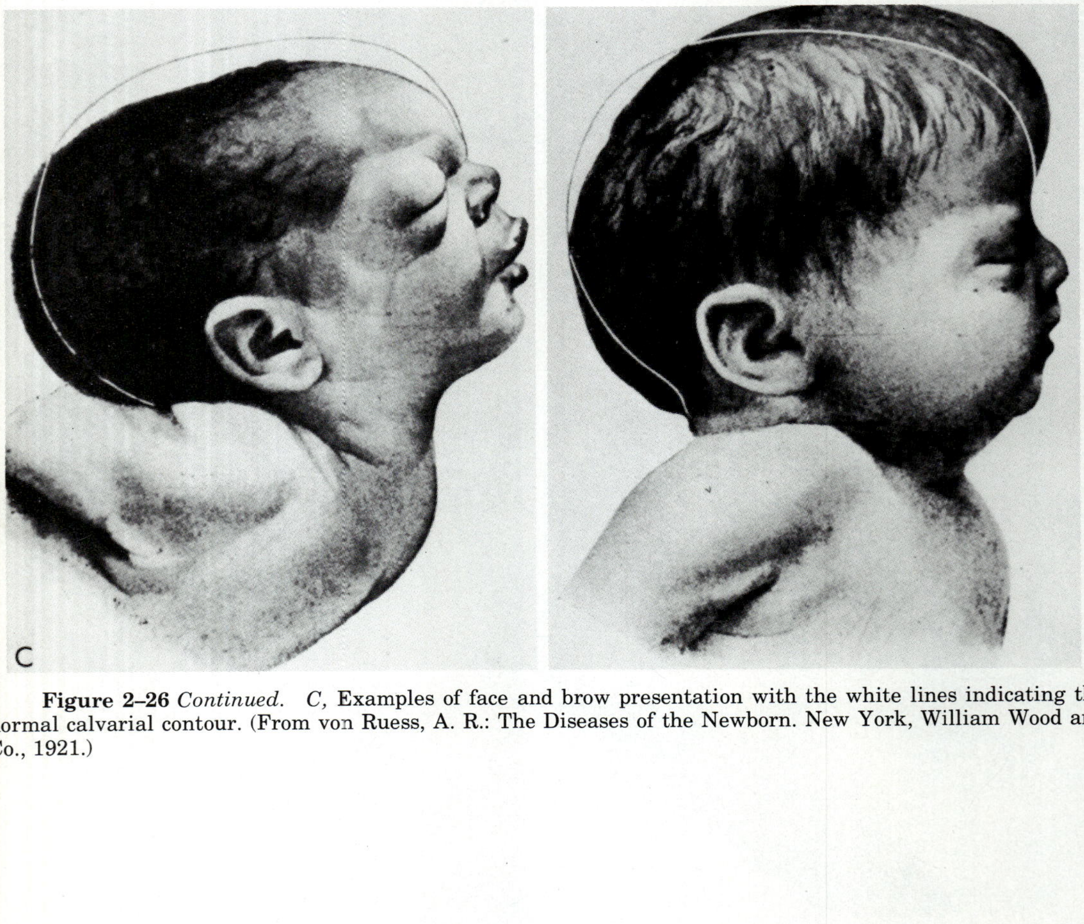

Figure 2–26 *Continued.* *C,* Examples of face and brow presentation with the white lines indicating the normal calvarial contour. (From von Ruess, A. R.: The Diseases of the Newborn. New York, William Wood and Co., 1921.)

17. SMALL UTERINE CAVITY DEFORMATION

Malformed Uterus, Uterine Fibroid(s), Small Uterus

GENESIS. Several different problems may limit the size and/or shape of the uterus and thus enhance the likelihood of fetal deformation. Examples include a malformed uterus, most commonly bicornuate or unicornuate. It is estimated that 1 to 2 per cent of women have a malformation of the uterus and that the general risk of a deformation problem for the fetus in a malformed uterus is 30 per cent.[1] This would imply that three to six infants per 1000 have a deformation problem secondary to being gestated in a malformed uterus. Rarely, a large uterine fibroid may be the cause. Sometimes a small fibroma may enlarge rapidly under the increased levels of estrogen during gestation. The small uterine cavity may result in miscarriage, stillbirth, or prematurity. It may also constrain the fetus and cause deformational problems.

FEATURES. All gradations of deformation of craniofacies, limbs, and thorax may occur, including overall constraint of fetal growth. The constraint of thoracic growth may be sufficient to impair lung growth and full morphogenesis. Hence, some of these infants have had respiratory distress at birth due to incomplete lung development.

MANAGEMENT, PROGNOSIS, AND COUNSEL. Insufficient uterine space for fetal growth should be considered as one possible explanation when a history of multiple miscarriages, stillbirths, prematurity, and/or serious deformation problems is obtained. Such findings may lead to the detection of a bicornuate uterus. Surgical improvement of the uterine size, if indicated and possible, will often bring about a great improvement in the chances of rearing a normal fetus to a term birth. Large uterine fibroids may also merit consideration of surgical intervention.

If the infant born of a small uterine cavity has respiratory distress, all efforts should be utilized to maintain oxygenation. If the infant can survive the early neonatal period, the prognosis is usually good to excellent.

If dislocation of the hip is present, it obviously merits management. Recurrence risk counsel depends on the cause of the problem of limited uterine space for fetal growth. The risk could be quite high and might be appreciably reduced by attempts to improve the uterine space.

DIFFERENTIAL DIAGNOSIS. A history of multiple miscarriages, stillbirths, and "malformed offspring" may lead to a consideration of chromosomal studies of parents and offspring, in search of a balanced chromosomal translocation in one of the parents, with consequent unbalanced zygotes. Limited uterine space should also be considered in such situations, especially since it may be possible to improve the uterine situation by surgery in some instances. A careful assessment of the infants born from a small uterine cavity who are considered "malformed" will indicate that they have multiple *deformations* rather than malformations.

REFERENCE

1. Miller, M.E., Dunn, P.M., and Smith, D.W.: Uterine malformation and fetal deformation. J. Pediatr. *94*:387, 1979.

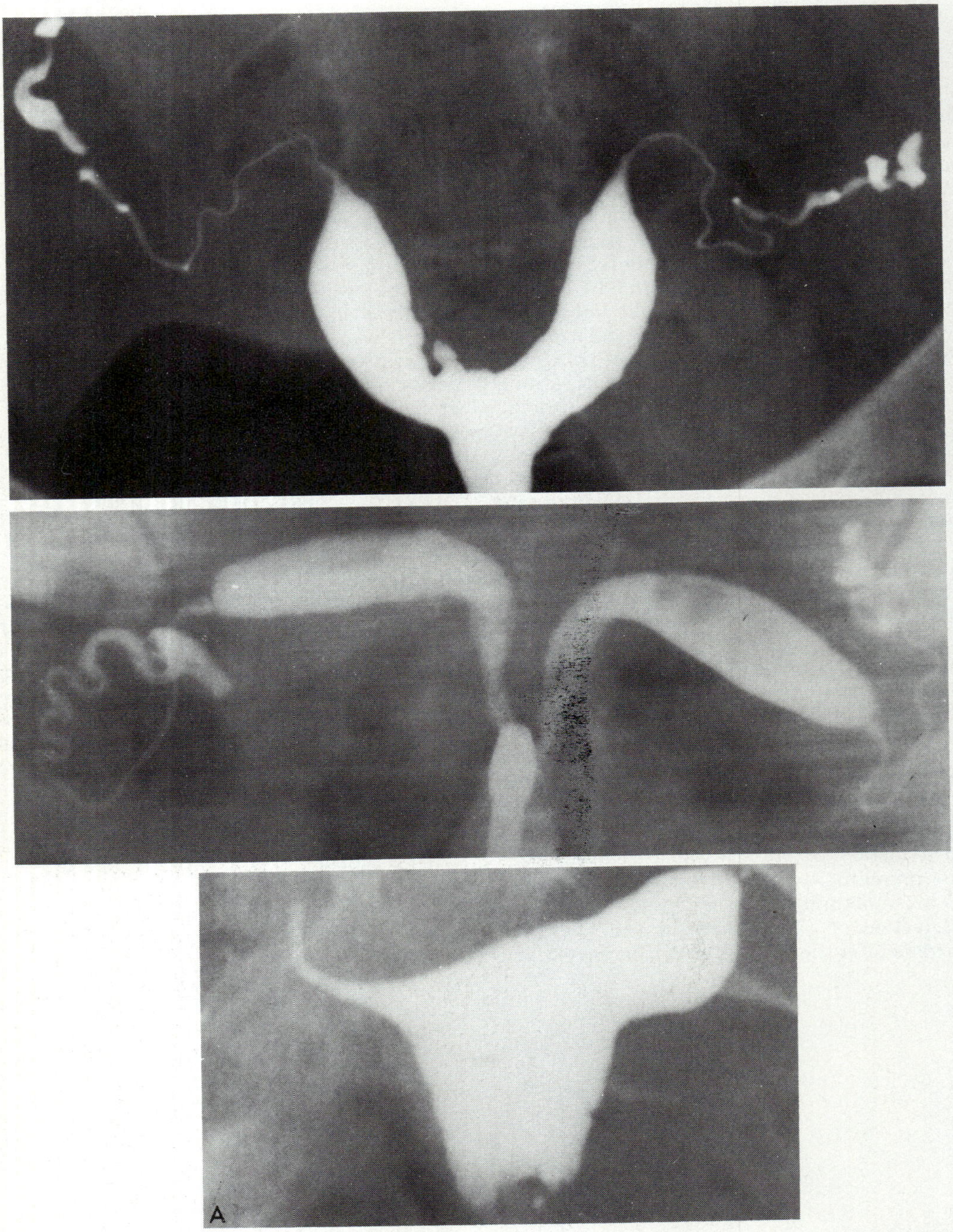

Figure 2–27. Small uterine cavity deformation. A, Three gradations of bicornuate uterus shown by hysterosalpingogram, each responsible for a deformational problem in the offspring.

Illustration continued on opposite page

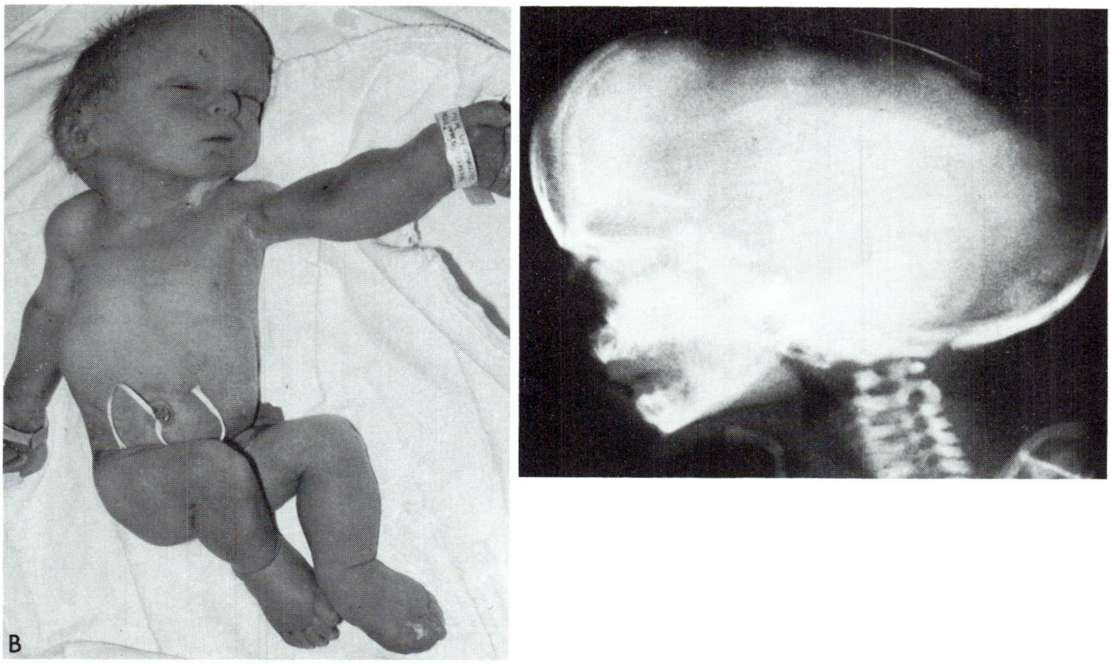

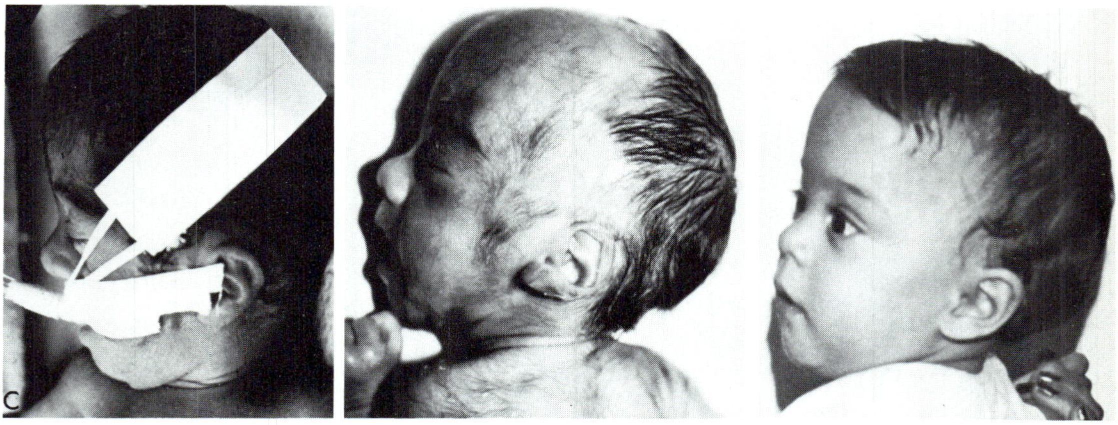

Figure 2–27 *Continued.* *B,* Severely deformed newborn infant gestated in a bicornuate uterus who died of respiratory insufficiency due to constraint induced lung hypoplasia. The proximal constraint of limb has resulted in distal lymphedema, and the head has been molded out of alignment in such a manner as to give the impression of low placed ears. The mother had a history of five previous miscarriages. (From Miller, M. E., Dunn, P. M., and Smith, D. W.: Uterine malformation and fetal deformation. J. Pediatr. *94*:387, 1979.) *C,* Prematurely born (34 week) infant with compressed craniofacies which initially had raised questions as to coronal craniostenosis. Within three weeks (middle) the face had grown forward and the question of craniostenosis was resolved. The right photo shows the infant at one year of age. (Courtesy of Dr. Kenneth Lyons Jones, University of California, San Diego. From Miller, M. E., Dunn, P. M., and Smith, D. W.: Uterine malformation and fetal deformation. J. Pediatr. *94*:387, 1979.)

Illustration continued on following page

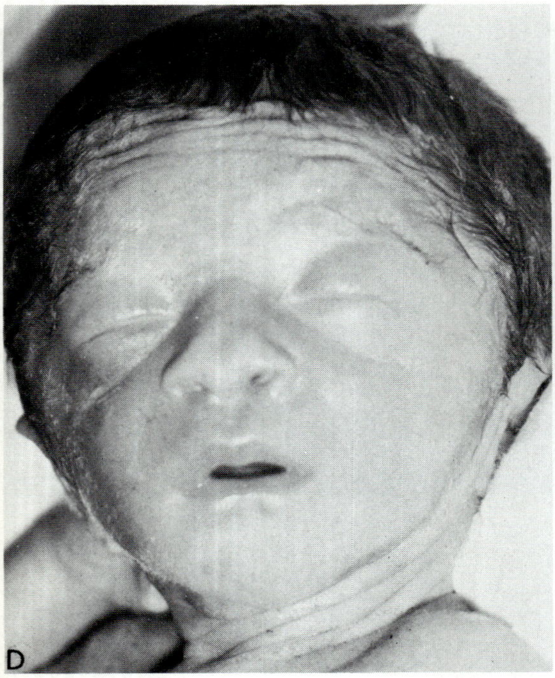

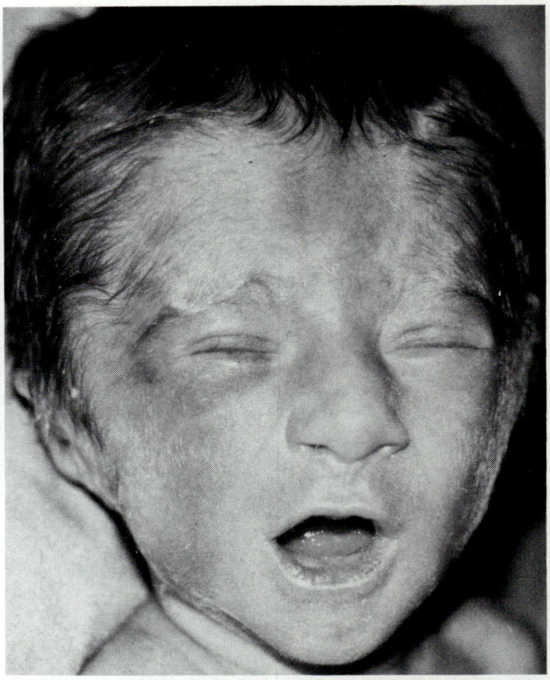

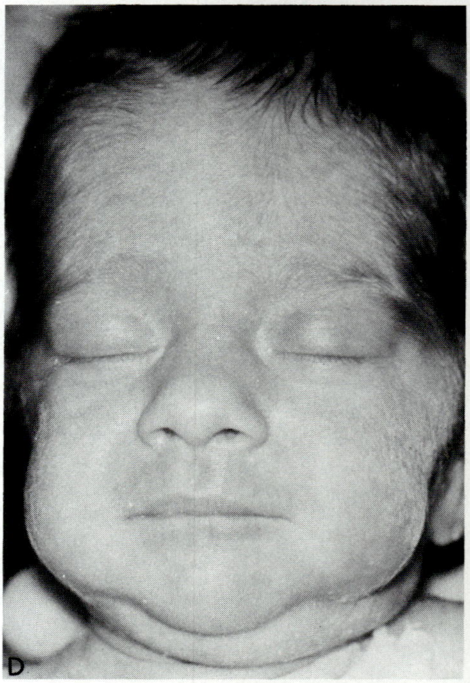

Figure 2–27 *Continued.* *D,* Prematurely born (34 week) infant gestated in a bicornuate uterus showing compressed facies with redundant skin. Follow-up at 48 hours and at 32 days shows the return toward normal form.

18. OLIGOHYDRAMNIOS SEQUENCE

GENESIS. The relative and absolute amount of amniotic fluid tends to decrease during the last trimester as the fetus is filling out the uterine cavity, as shown in Figure 2–28*A*. A serious deficiency of amniotic fluid will yield unusual uterine constraint. In early fetal life this deficiency may be secondary to amniotic rupture and may be accompanied by constrictive and disruptive bands and strands of amnion. The consequences of very early rupture with amniotic band disruptions can be horrendous and may include compressive consequences of early constraint, including scoliosis and even incomplete limb morphogenesis. These early cases are most commonly lethal and are found predominantly in spontaneous abortuses. Later rupture of the amnion may or may not be accompanied by amniotic bands. If later bands are present, they are usually limited to constrictive bands around various parts of one or more limbs. Chronic leakage of amniotic fluid, usually two to three or more weeks before delivery, is one cause of the oligohydramnios sequence (Figure 2–28*B*).

Oligohydramnios may occur with maternal hypertension, severe toxemia, placental insufficiency, and postmaturity, although the precise reason is unknown. It may also occur in one of monozygotic twins because of a placental vascular shunt. If one twin is transfusing the other, the donor tends to be hypovolemic with reduced renal blood flow, the presumed reason for the oligohydramnios.

Oligohydramnios may also be caused by a lack of adequate urine flow into the amniotic space because of a fetal malformation. The most common cause is renal agenesis but it may also be due to polycystic kidneys or to urethral obstruction. By the twentieth to twenty-fifth week of gestation urine becomes a major constituent of amniotic fluid. Hence, oligohydramnios is predominantly a feature of these urinary tract malformations during the last trimester of gestation. Idiopathic oligohydramnios may also occur, but is rare.

FEATURES. The features of the oligohydramnios sequence often include those of the breech deformation type, since about 50 per cent of these infants are in breech position at birth. As Smithells has aptly stated: "The fetus is in drydock and cannot maneuver for delivery."[2]

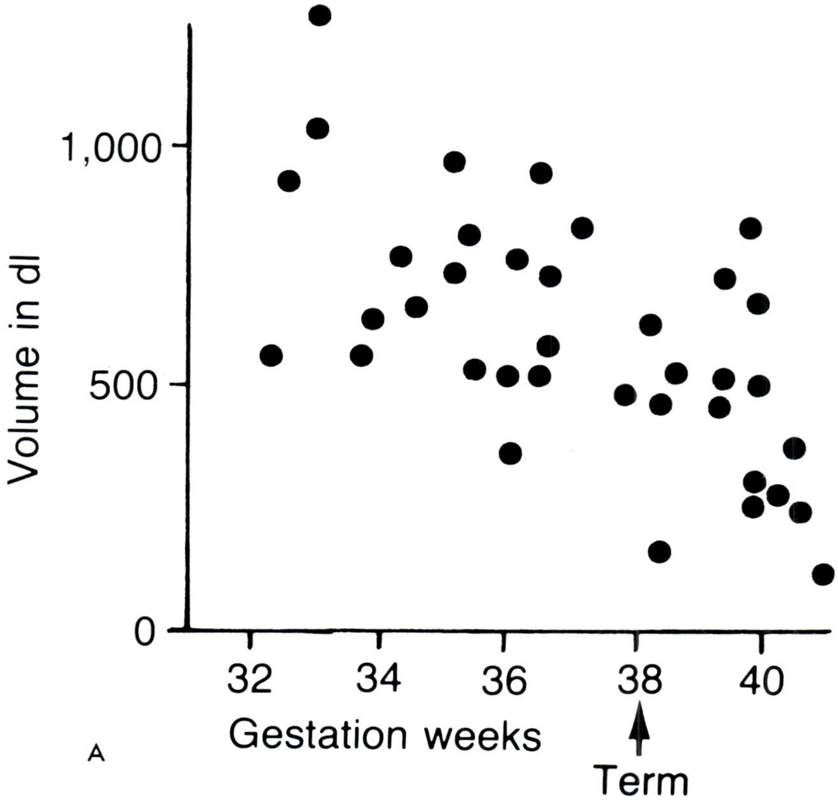

Figure 2–28. Oligohydramnios deformation sequence. *A*, Progressive decrease in volume of amniotic fluid during the last trimester.

Illustration continued on following page

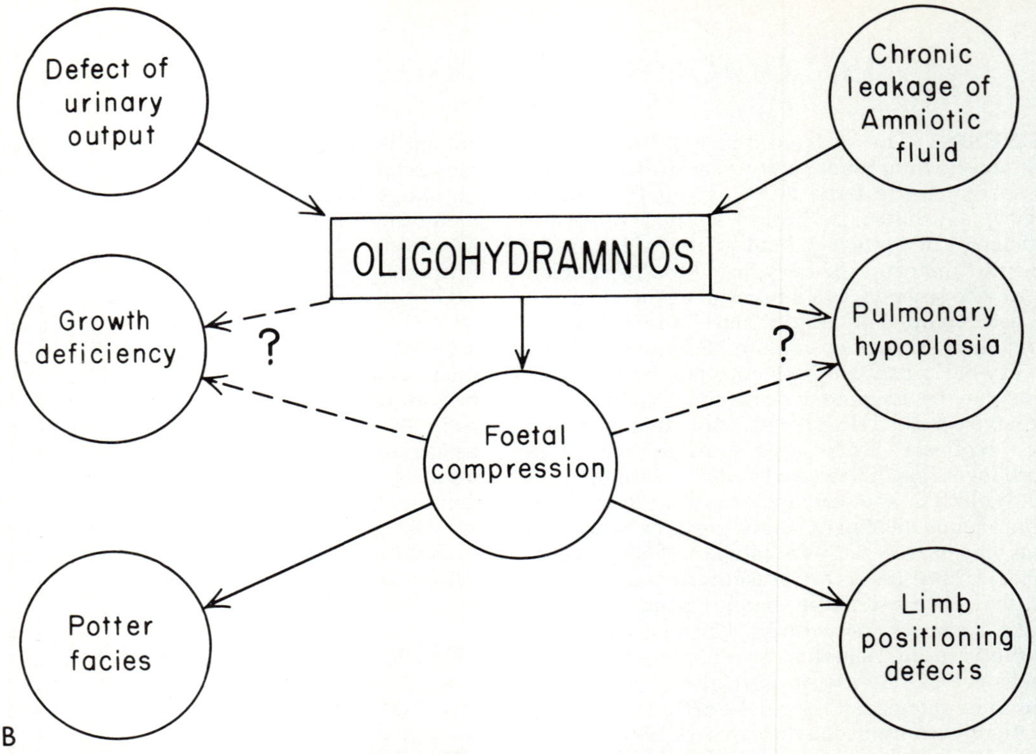

Figure 2–28 *Continued.* *B,* Origins and impact of oligohydramnios on the fetus.

Illustration continued on opposite page

Craniofacial. The head usually looks as though a silk stocking had been pulled down over it, causing a flattened nose and flattened or "accordioned" external ears.

Limbs. The hands and feet — especially the feet — tend to be in aberrant position, often with stiffness of the joints, which have been limited in their mobility. The hips may be dislocated.

Thorax and Lung. Thoracic growth is restrained, and the full growth and maturation of the lung is thwarted.[1] The lungs often do not progress beyond a four to five month level of development and hence may be deficient or lacking in surfactant and be incapable of aerobic expansion and/or oxygen exchange. This respiratory insufficiency is the most common cause of demise in the early postnatal period. Not uncommonly attempts to resuscitate the newborn baby lead to pneumothorax, a frequent complication in the baby with respiratory insufficiency due to oligohydramnios.

Skin. The skin tends to be redundant, presumably the result of overgrowth related to external constraint. This gives rise to accentuated inner canthal and infraorbital skin folds, which contribute to the "Potter" facies and sometimes may yield the impression of a web neck.

Other. Concretions of amnion cells may build up on the relatively dry surface of the placenta, a feature termed amnion nodosa.

MANAGEMENT, PROGNOSIS, AND COUNSEL. If the oligohydramnios is due to renal agenesis or another type of severe renal problem, attempts to artificially oxygenate the neonate are of little or no value. However, if the deficit of amniotic fluid is due to chronic leakage of amniotic fluid, then every attempt toward oxygenation should be pursued, since the renal function is normal. If such an infant survives, there is usually catch-up growth with a restitution toward normal form. The recurrence risk relates to the basic problem that gave rise to the oligohydramnios. Thus, with chronic leakage of fluid the recurrence risk would be very low, with defects such as urethral obstruction or renal agenesis the risk may be several per cent, and with some types of polycystic kidney the risk may be as high as 25 per cent (autosomal recessive).

DIFFERENTIAL DIAGNOSIS. See *Genesis.*

REFERENCES

1. Thomas, I.T., and Smith, D.W.: Oligohydramnios, cause of the non-renal features of Potter's syndrome, including pulmonary hypoplasia. J. Pediatr. *84*:811, 1974.
2. Scott, J.S.: The volume and circulation of the liquor amnii: Clinical observations. Proc. Roy. Soc. Med. *59*:1128, 1966.

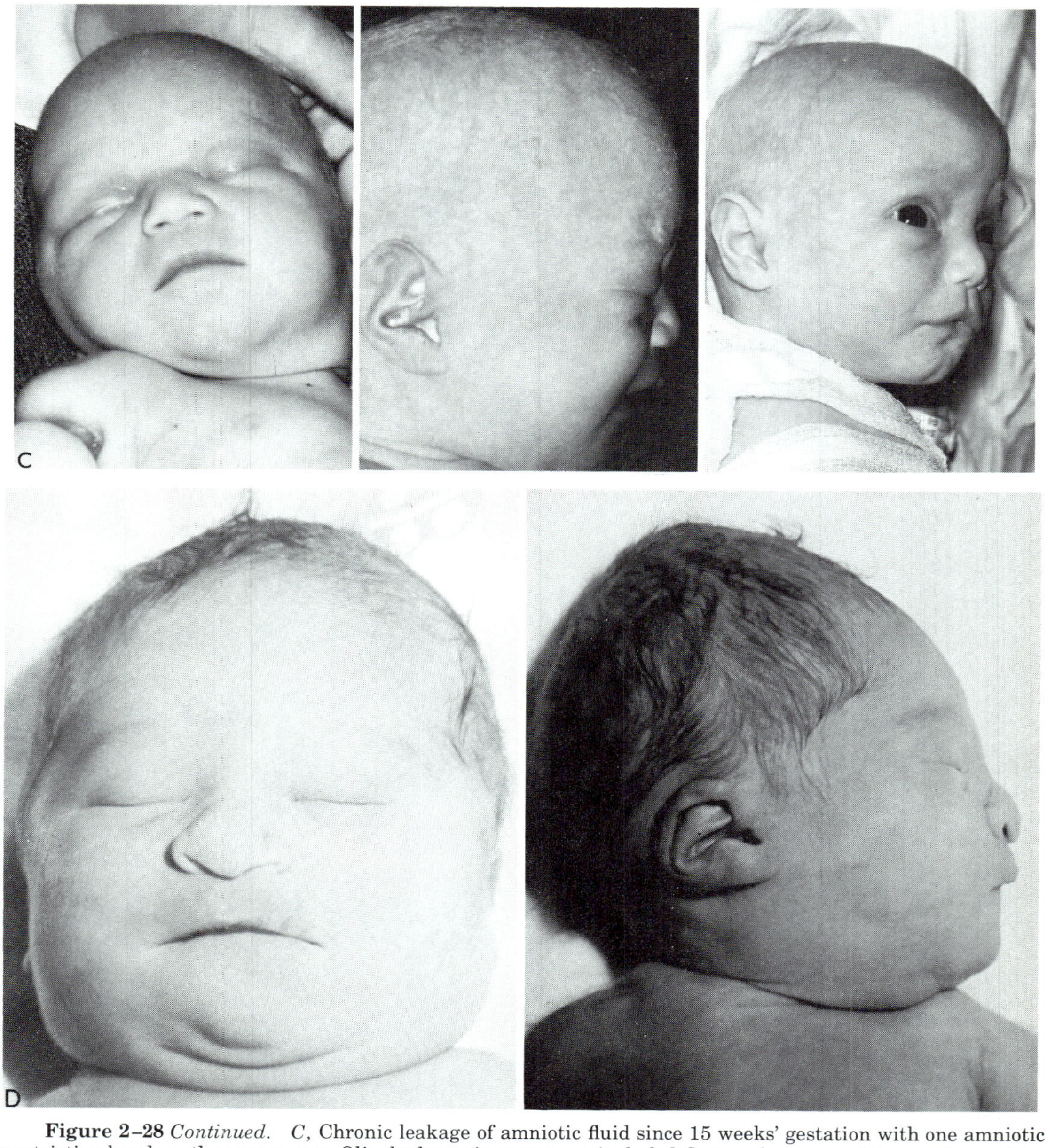

Figure 2–28 *Continued.* *C,* Chronic leakage of amniotic fluid since 15 weeks' gestation with one amniotic constrictive band on the upper arm. Oligohydramnios sequence included flattened nose, auricle, and loose skin. Oxygenation was maintained for transient respiratory insufficiency, and the infant returned toward normal form by six weeks (right). *D,* Compressed facies, redundant skin, and accordion ear of a newborn infant with severe oligohydramnios secondary to renal agenesis.

Illustration continued on following page

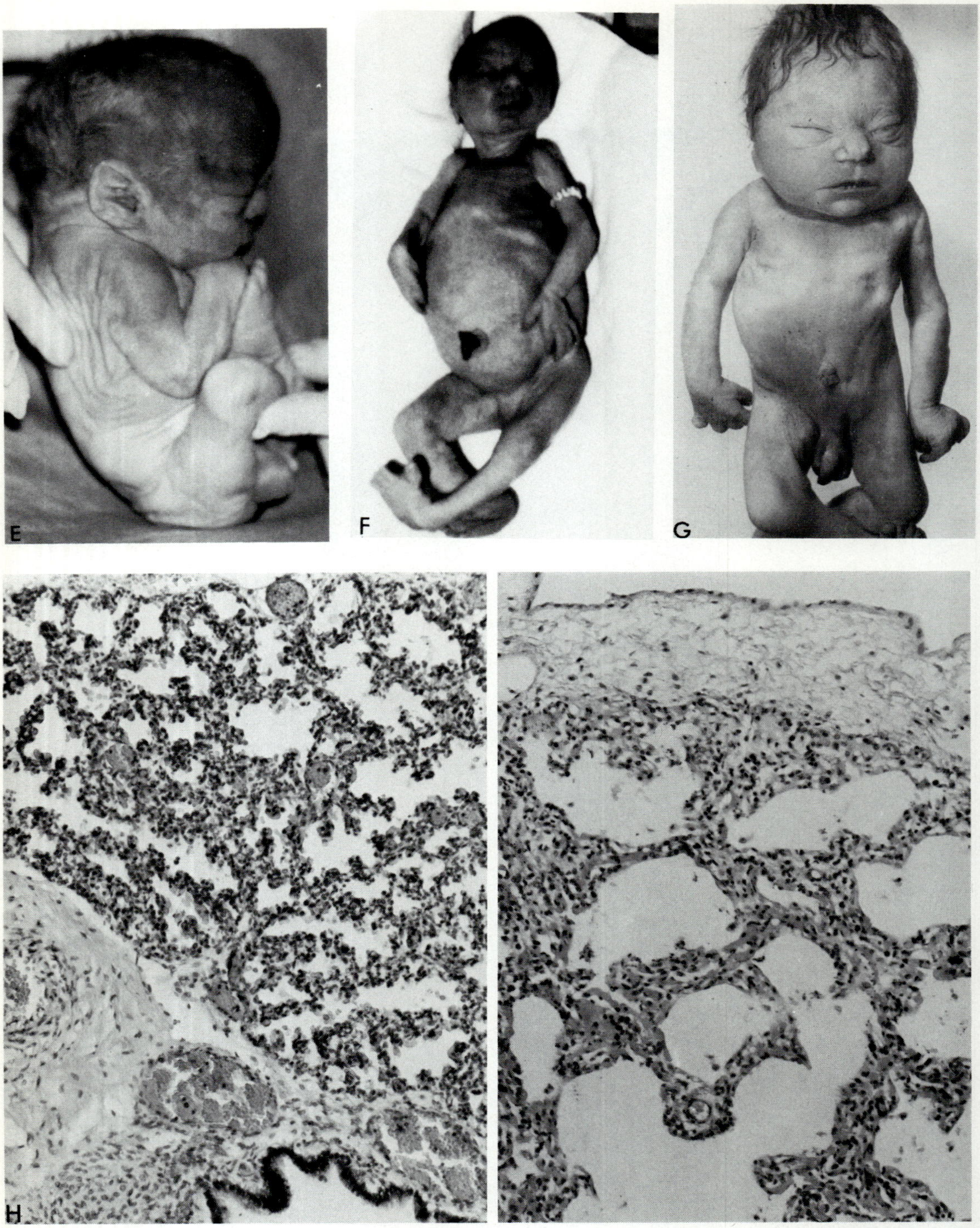

Figure 2–28 *Continued.* *E,* Oligohydramnios deformation sequence plus breech sequence, including "breech head" in an infant with renal agenesis. Note the redundant skin. *F,* Oligohydramnios sequence with severe deficit of thoracic growth and limb deformation in an infant with massive polycystic kidneys that have distended the abdomen. *G,* Renal agenesis with severe oligohydramnios. Note the effects not only on the limbs but also on the thoracic cage. *H,* Lung hypoplasia secondary to severe oligohydramnios yielding non-expansile lung with limited aerobic exchange, in contrast to normal lung (right). (From Thomas, I. T., and Smith, D. W.: Oligohydramnios, cause of the non-renal features of Potter's syndrome. J. Pediatr. *84*:811, 1974.)

19. EXTRAUTERINE PREGNANCY

GENESIS, FEATURES, PROGNOSIS. In rare instances fertilization of the ovum may take place outside the fallopian tube, and the zygote may then implant outside of the uterus. When this occurs the conceptus seldom survives. Oligohydramnios is frequent. If survival does occur there is likely to be severe constraint of fetal development. One child who survived an abdominal pregnancy, and who was described as being "the worst looking newborn I have ever seen," after birth returned to normal appearance.

REFERENCE

1. Scott, J.S.: The volume and circulation of the liquor amnii: Clinical observations. Proc. Roy. Soc. Med. *59*:1128, 1966.

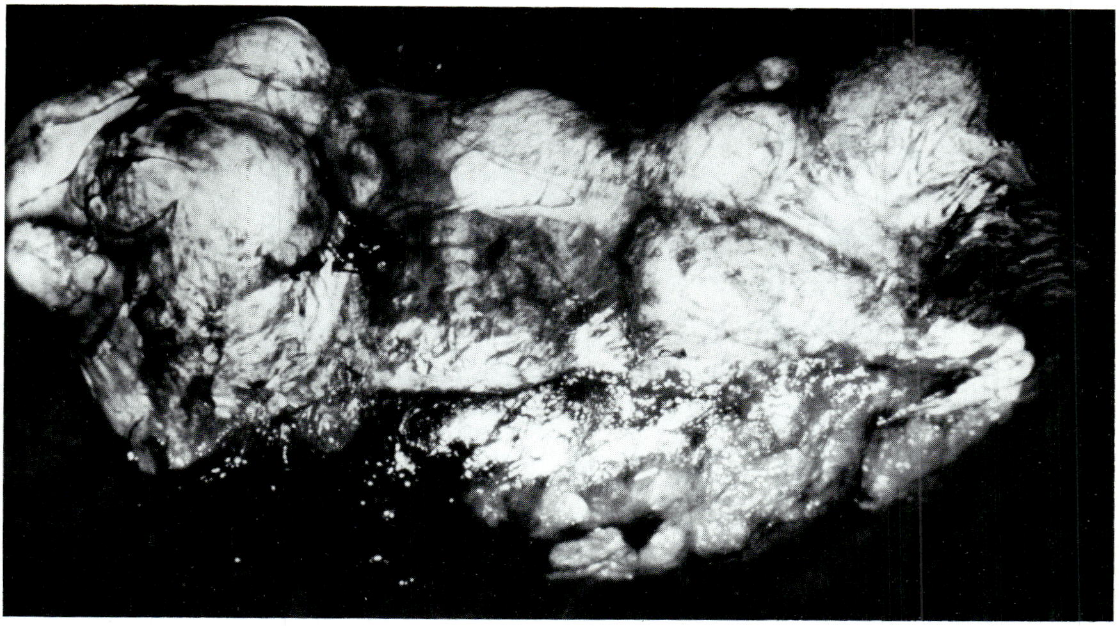

Figure 2–29. Extrauterine pregnancy. Extrauterine pregnancy showing intact amniotic sac which contains no amniotic fluid and encases the compressed fetus. (Courtesy of Dr. Scott, Department of Obstetrics and Gynecology, Leeds, England.)

20. EARLY CONSTRAINT DEFECTS

Constraint that occurs during the latter period of gestation usually causes molded deformations with good prospects for spontaneous or assisted return to normal form. However, constraint that occurs in early morphogenesis can have more severe and lasting impacts on form. The type of defects that can be produced by constraint within the first trimester fall into three categories, as summarized in Table 2–6.

All three types of defects were experimentally produced by Poswillo[1] by early amniotic sac rupture in rat embryos of 15½ days' gestation. At that time the rat embryo is at about the same stage as the human is at six to seven weeks of gestation. The mesenchymal condensations of the limb bones have occurred, but the fingers are not fully separated. The lip is fused, but the palatal shelves have yet to close. Following rupture of the amnion, the animals were found to be compressed in a cephalocaudal fashion with the developing mandible thrust against the sternum and the limbs in various stages of compression. Table 2–7 summarizes the frequency of the three types of defects observed in the 32 animals so treated.[1] There were no defects in the control animals. All animals showed a small jaw, caused by compression of the mandible against the sternum. In all but one fetus this had caused the tongue to be maintained between the palatal shelves and thereby prevented closure of the palatal shelves. The failure of full separation of the fingers (syndactyly) was also interpreted as incomplete morphogenesis secondary to compression. The loss of the radius, the femur, and major limb parts, which must have been normally present at the time of the induced compression, was interpreted as the result of focal compressive necrosis with disruptive defects via compressive oligohydramnios in the rodent. Poswillo has shown that the compression leads to edema and hemorrhage with tissue damage and resorption.

We are only beginning to appreciate comparable defects in man as presumed consequences of early compression in utero. Among the patients with early rupture of the amnion who have amniotic bands (bands were also present in 19 per cent of the rats in Poswillo's study) we have observed talipes deformations, syndactyly, and limb reductions of a type that could not be readily explained by amniotic band constrictions. Among the amniotic band cases that must have occurred in early development we have also observed scoliosis and other deformations. We have also observed instances of the Robin malformation sequence, formerly termed Pierre Robin syndrome, in which the total findings were compatible with a constraint causation for the early micrognathia and a secondary posterior cleft palate caused by obstruction of palatine closure by the tongue. Poswillo[1] found that 29 per cent of his rat fetuses with the Robin sequence defects induced by oligohydramnios compression also had limb defects, most commonly deformational in type. Dunn[3] states that half of his human patients with Robin sequence defects had deformations, especially of the limb. Hanson and Smith[4] report that 11 per cent of their patients in whom Robin sequence was part of a known syndrome also had limb defects.

We have also observed early limb compressive effects of all three types (Table 2–6) in individuals who had been reared in a constrictive bicornuate uterus (four cases) and one reared in a uterus that contained a 10 cm fibroid.[5] Matsunaga and Shiota[6] also have recognized early spatial limitation as a factor in constraint induced malformation. They found that 11.6 per cent of 43 embryos and fetuses recovered from ectopic tubal pregnancies had structural defects, as did 6.2 per cent of 97 fetuses from myomatous pregnancies, in contrast to 3.3 per cent structural defects among 3474 normally implanted therapeutic abortuses from non-myomatous uteri. Two of the

Table 2–6. Types of Defects Produced in Early Gestation by Constraint

1. *Molded Deformations:* Similar to those produced in late fetal life, but often more severe and difficult to return to normal form because of early onset.
2. *Incomplete Morphogenesis:* The constraint may limit or prevent full completion of a normal stage in morphogenesis.
3. *Disruption of Morphogenesis:* The constraint may cause edema, hemorrhage and focal necrosis with loss of previously formed tissue.

Table 2–7. Defects Found by Poswillo[1] in 32 Rat Fetuses Following Oligohydramnios Compression at 15 1/2 Days (similar to 42–45 days in human)

1. Molded Deformations	100%
a. Micrognathia	100%
b. Talipes	5%
2. Incomplete Morphogenesis	97%
a. Failure of palatine closure	97%
b. Syndactyly	9%
3. Disruption of Morphogenesis	12%
a. Absent radius, femur	6%
b. Phocomelia	6%

five with structural defects who were reared in the fallopian tube had amelia.

Our knowledge of the impact of early in-utero constraint in the human is just beginning to grow. The future findings should be of interest. We recently observed an instance of early neurapraxia with apparent permanent impact on growth and function of the affected limb.

REFERENCES

1. Poswillo, D.: Observations of fetal posture and causal mechanisms of congenital deformity of the palate, mandible and limbs. J. Dent. Res. *45*(3): 583, 1966.
2. Kennedy, L.A., and Persaud, T.V.N.: Pathogenesis of developmental defects induced in the rat by amniotic sac puncture. Acta Anat. (Basel) *97*:23, 1977.
3. Dunn, P.M.: The influence of the intrauterine environment in the causation of congenital postural deformities, with special reference to congenital dislocation of the hip. (Thesis for MD degree) University of Cambridge, 1969.
4. Hanson, J.W., and Smith, D.W.: U-shaped palatal defect in the Robin anomalad: Developmental and clinical relevance. J. Pediatr. *87*:30, July, 1975.
5. Graham, J.M., Jr., Miller, M.E., Stephan, M.J., and Smith, D.W.: Limb reduction anomalies and early in-utero limb compression. J. Pediatr., *96*:1052, 1980.
6. Matsunaga, E., and Shiota, K.: Ectopic pregnancy and myoma uteri: Teratogenic effects and maternal characteristics. Teratology, in press.

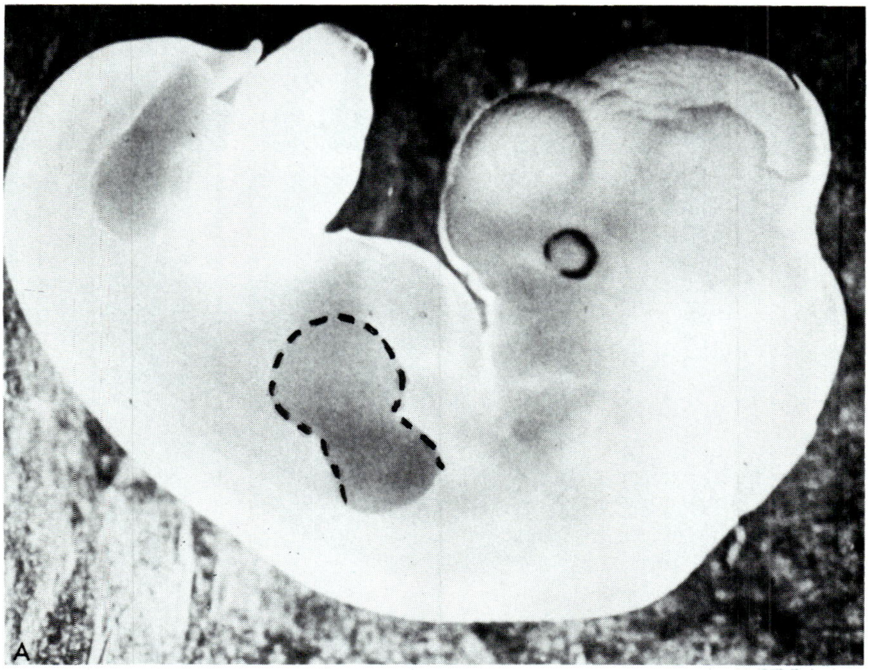

Figure 2–30. Early constraint defects. *A*, Human embryo at about 42 days of development with hand plate formed (outlined) but no separation of the finger rays. It is around this era that constraint of the developing limb has been shown in animal studies to cause edema, hemorrhage, and resorptive necrosis with loss of previously normal tissues. The process of separation of the digits may also be impaired, yielding syndactyly.

Illustration continued on following page

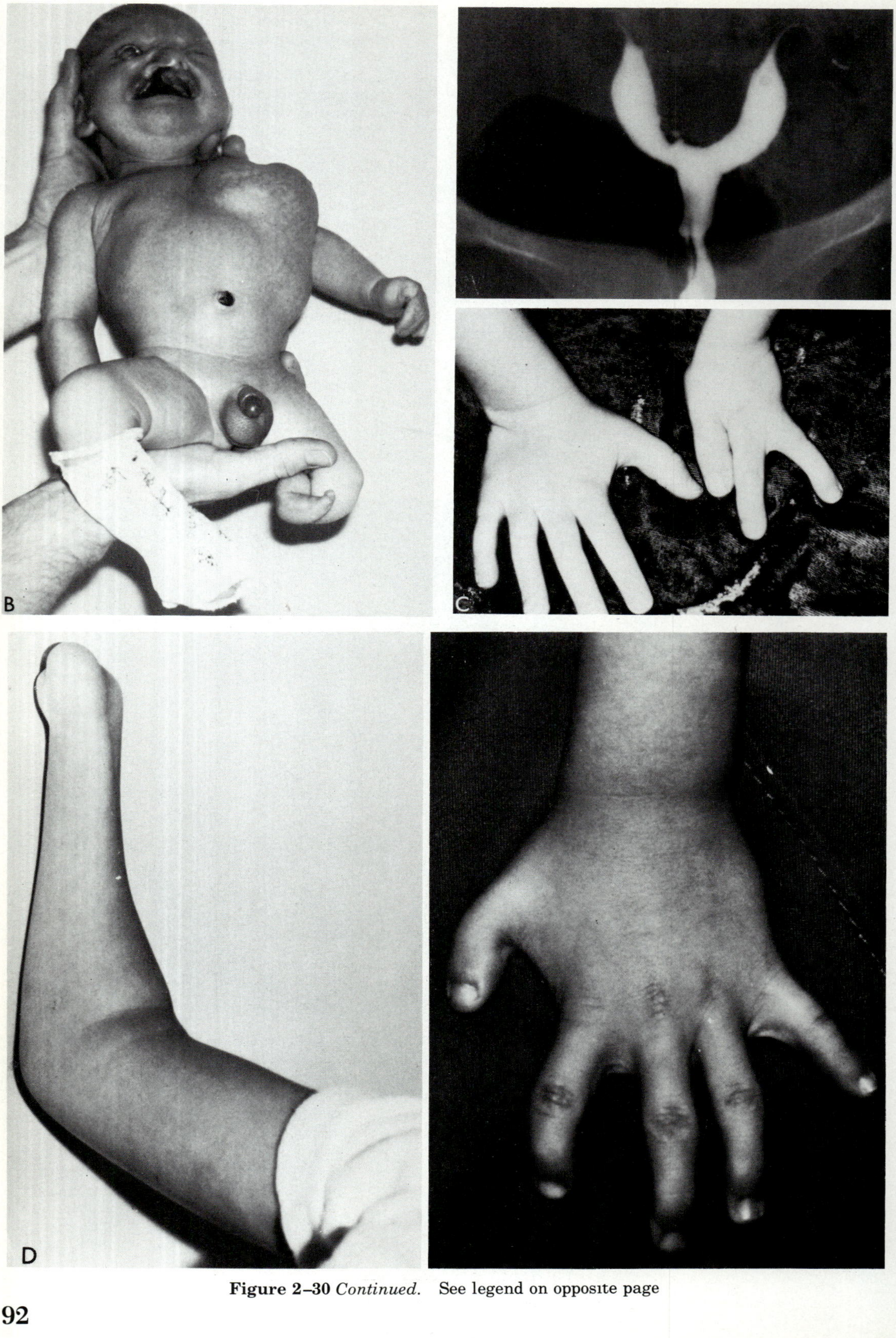

Figure 2–30 *Continued.* See legend on opposite page

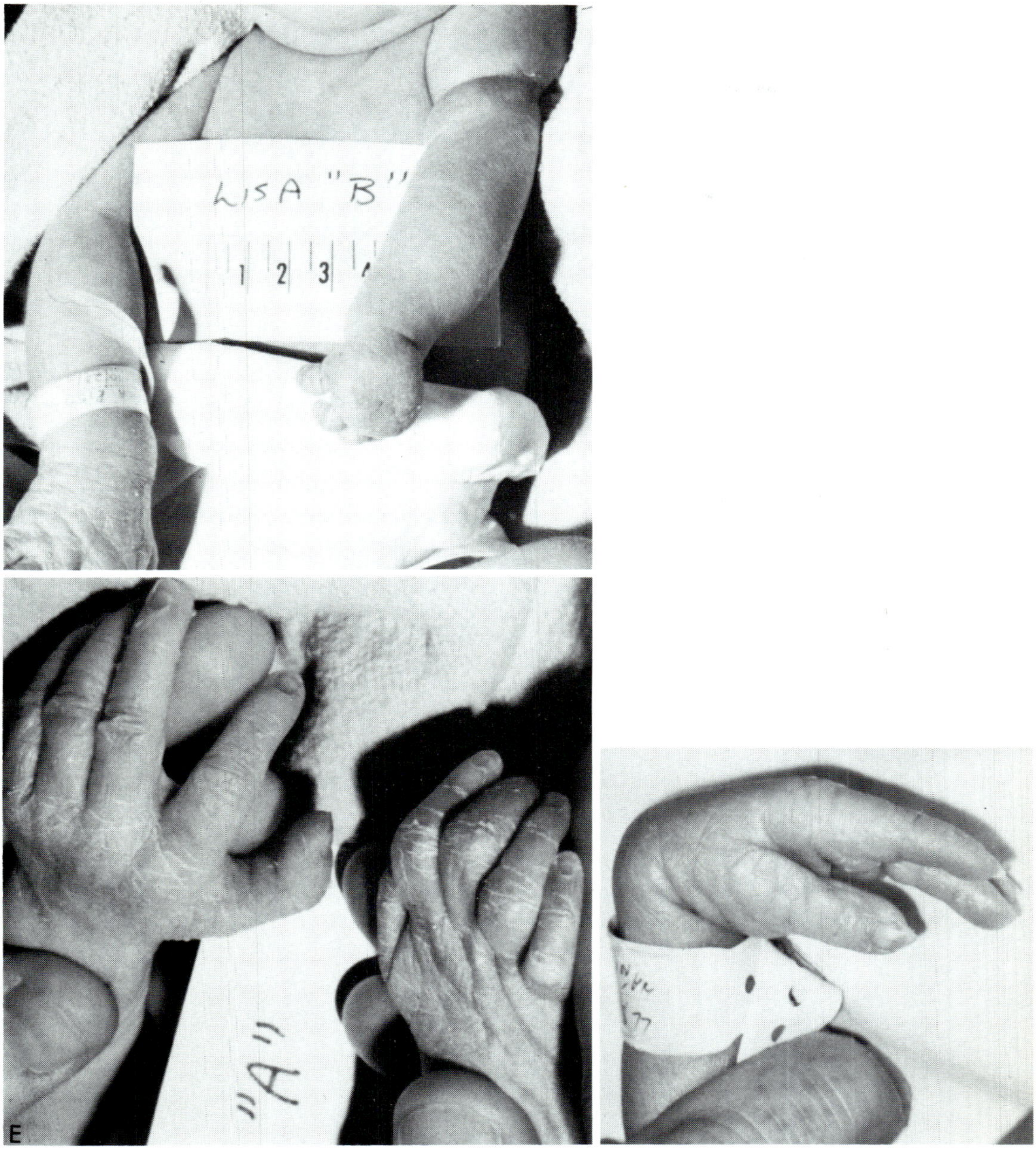

Figure 2–30 *Continued.* *B,* Infant with consequences of presumed early rupture of the amnion with amniotic band disruption of right facies including eye, tethered disruption of left thoracic cage, and band constrictions on left thumb. In addition, there is partial limb reduction of the left lower limb and failure of separation of the left second and third fingers, presumed effects of the early constraint at the time of amnion rupture. *C,* Unilateral oligodactyly (B) in a child reared in the above bicornuate uterus (A). *D,* Lack of distal arm (A) and contralateral hypoplasia of thumb and mild second to third finger syndactyly (B) in a child reared in a bicornuate uterus. *E,* Monozygotic, monoamniotic twins with early rupture of amnion leading to amniotic band with distal arm and hand hypoplasia in twin B, while twin A has a unilateral Erb's palsy with small arm on the affected side. This neurological deficit was interpreted as the consequence of constraint of the arm against the chest yielding a radial nerve palsy at the time of the temporary oligohydramnios caused by early amnion rupture. Courtesy of Dr. J. Alan MacFarlane, Fairbanks, Alaska. (*B, C,* and *D* from Graham, J. M., Jr., Miller, M. E., Stephan, M. J., and Smith, D. W.: Limb reduction anomalies and early in-utero limb compression. J. Pediatr. *96*:1052, 1980.)

21. POSTNATAL DEFORMATION

PREMATURE INFANT. The liability toward deformation depends on the magnitude and duration of the forces applied and the pliability of the host. The prematurely born infant is more malleable than the term baby. In addition, the premature is more hypotonic and is more likely to lie in one position more persistently. If the surface on which he or she is lying is relatively firm, the premature infant will often develop flattening on both sides of the head, with a scaphocephalic, narrow head shape. In similar fashion, the thoracic cage may become relatively narrow in the anterior-posterior diameter.

These subtle deformities are largely preventable by utilizing soft and easily malleable surfaces, such as a water bed, for the premature baby to lie on.

The premature baby may persistently lie on one particular side of the head and can develop a significant oblique-shaped (plagiocephalic) head as a result.

FULL TERM INFANT. A term infant with a neurological deficiency or who is seriously neglected may tend to lie in one position and may develop asymmetric flattening of one side of the head.

Torticollis may develop postnatally, especially when there has been stretch injury to the sternocleidomastoid muscle at birth.

Thumb sucking seldom causes deformation in early infancy. However, once the teeth have developed, thumb sucking can deform the upper jaw. This is especially true when the child "pulls" out on the teeth.

Growth of the mandible tends to catch up to that of the maxilla during the first few years, and the mandibular teeth and mandible normally conform to the maxillary teeth. Supernumerary teeth or absence of teeth can lead to mild deformation, including malocclusions between the maxilla and mandible. Nowhere have the principles of mechanical treatment been more effectively employed than in the mouth. Once the teeth have fully erupted, they may be utilized as anchors for a variety of devices to alter the growth and/or alignment of the maxilla and/or mandible. Intraoral devices that provide rather small pressures on developing teeth can have a considerable impact on form.

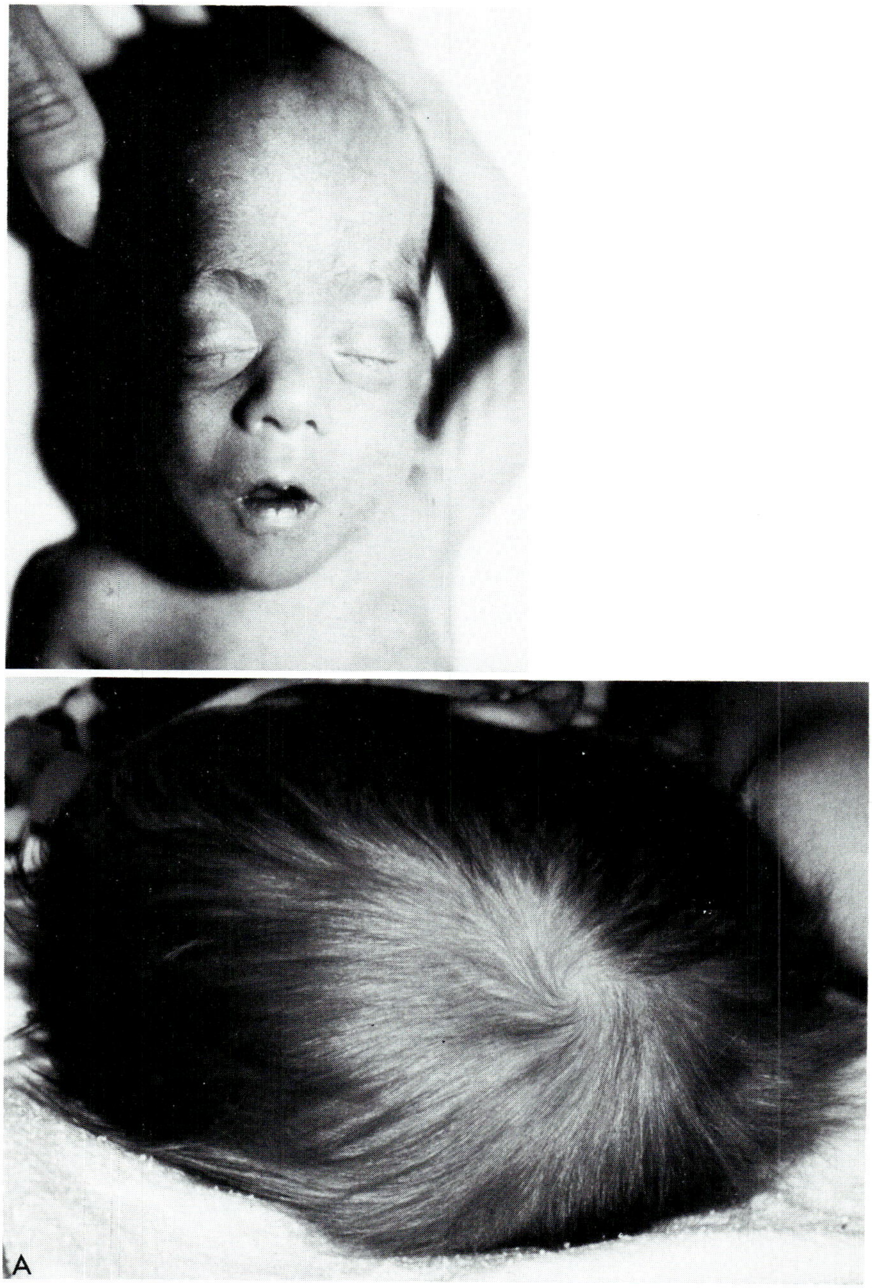

Figure 2–31. Postnatal deformation. *A*, Prematurely born infants with flattening of the head due to lying on relatively firm surfaces on one side of the head and then the other. Note that the impact is evident in the upper face as well.

Illustration continued on following page

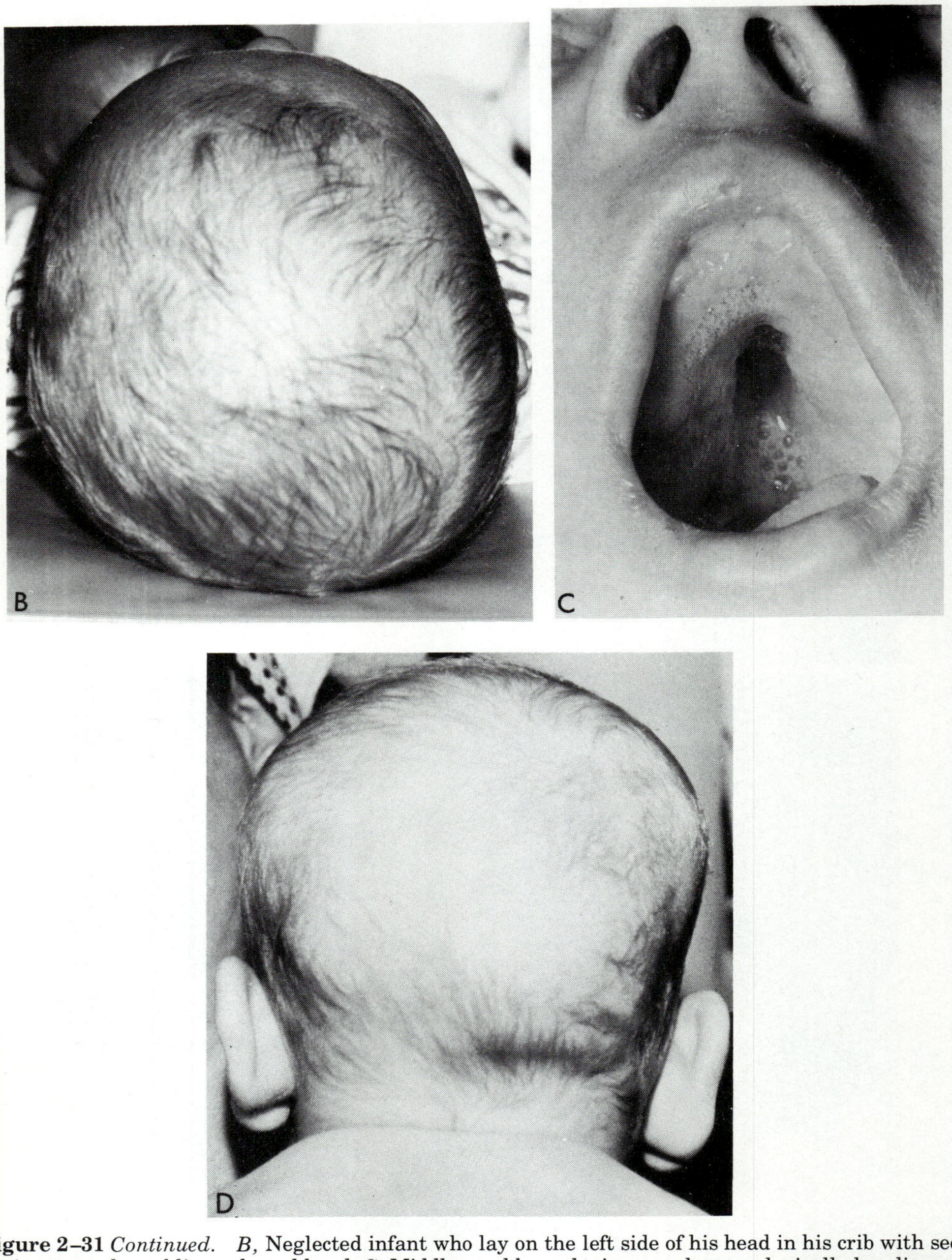

Figure 2–31 *Continued.* *B,* Neglected infant who lay on the left side of his head in his crib with secondary deformation toward an oblique shaped head. *C,* Middle-aged boy who is severely neurologically handicapped with a poor suck and swallow because of near-drowning at two years. Note the postnatal development of prominent lateral palatine ridges and a narrow palate, secondary to disuse. *D,* Impact of physical forces on the growth of auricle. This infant preferred to lie on the right side, and as a consequence the right ear was 0.5 cm longer than the left ear. (*C* and *D* courtesy Kenneth Lyons Jones, M.D., University of California at San Diego.)

Chapter Three

CLINICAL APPROACH TO DEFORMATION PROBLEMS

Mechanical forces are integral to morphogenesis, and unusual mechanical forces tend to yield unusual forms in developing tissues. The consequences are termed a deformation or deformation sequence.* The latter term refers to the manifold consequences of a single deforming cause, such as the oligohydramnios sequence. These types of defects are to be distinguished from malformations, in which there has been an intrinsic problem in the development of one or more tissues, and from disruptions, in which there has been a breakdown of a previously normal tissue.* This general classification of structural defects is summarized in Figure 3–1.

Given a structural defect which is presumed to be caused by aberrant mechanical forces, it is prudent to strive to determine whether the unusual forces were of extrinsic origin, affecting an otherwise normal fetus, or of intrinsic origin, resulting from a fetal problem such as a malformation. These two predominant modes of causation for deformation are shown in Figure 3–2. The distinction is based on a number of historical and physical findings. The major emphasis of this text is on extrinsic deformations due to in-utero constraint. Hence this category will be considered first, to be followed by the interaction of both extrinsic and intrinsic factors in the genesis of some deformations, and finally the intrinsic deformations due to a fetal malformation.

*The term sequence implicates the initiating defect plus its chain of consequences. For a malformation it implicates the initiating localized structural defect and any of its secondary consequences, some of which can be deformational. For a deformation it implicates the initiating *mechanical* aberration plus all of its secondary consequences. The word sequence was deemed more appropriate to convey this concept than the word syndrome (of which it may be a component) or anomalad or complex (synonymously utilized words in the past). Sequence was recommended for this usage by an international meeting on nomenclature organized by Professor Jürgen Spranger at the University of Mainz on November 10–12, 1979.

EXTRINSIC DEFORMATIONS DUE TO UTERINE CONSTRAINT

The presumption in this category is that there is no primary problem within the fetus, but that the deformations are secondary to extrinsic forces that have deformed an otherwise normal fetus. The most common cause of extrinsic deformation is *uterine constraint.* About 2 per cent of babies are born with an extrinsic deformation; hence these are relatively common problems.[1, 2]

There is usually an adequate amount of amniotic fluid to cushion the fetus and allow full growth and mobility prior to 36 to 37 weeks of gestation (from conception). Thus, as Harrison and Malpas[3] indicated, one of the functions of the amniotic fluid is to distend the uterus and enable the fetus to move freely, to develop, and to grow with equal pressure in all regions with no excessive or localized constraint. As the fetus becomes crowded in its uterine "sac" during late gestation it will usually settle into a position in which the largest mobile fetal parts, the relatively bulky legs, have ample room. Thus the fetus tends to assume the vertex presentation. The implication that many of the extrinsic deformations are pro-

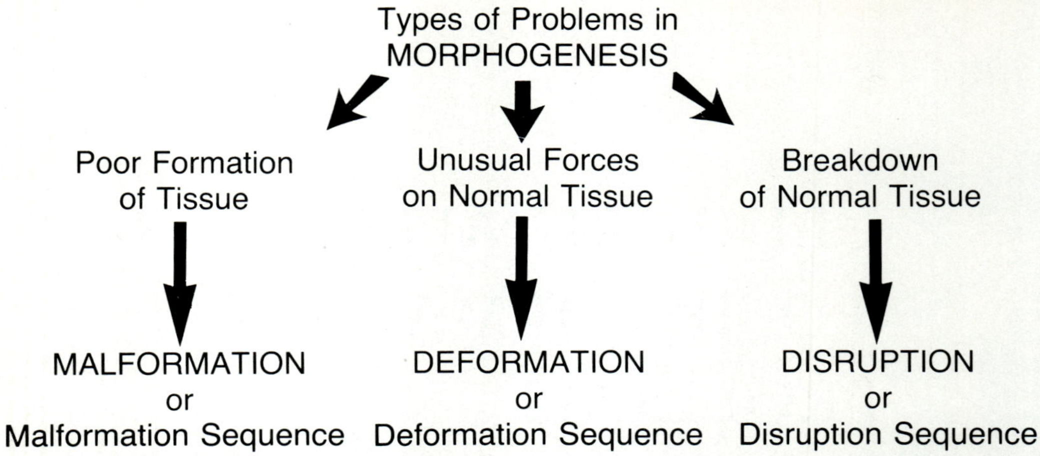

Figure 3–1. The three predominant types of problems in the developmental pathology of structural defects.

duced during late fetal life is supported by the observations of Nishimura,[4] who found that both dislocation of the hip and clubfoot are rare features in abortuses prior to 20 weeks of gestation.

After about 35 to 38 weeks of gestation, the human fetus tends to grow out of proportion to the uterine cavity, as is evident in viewing Figures 3–3 and 3–4. During this time the fetus is growing rapidly while the relative proportion of amniotic fluid is decreasing. The fetus thus becomes increasingly constrained. Uterine constraint of the rapidly growing malleable fetal tissues may result in mechanically induced deformations.

Since the cause of one deformation may often have led to other problems of constraint in the pliable fetus, there is a non-random occurrence of more than one deformation in the same child.[2] Dunn found that 30 per cent of newborn infants with a deformation problem had more than a single deformation. This non-random association of multiple deformations is summarized in Figure 3–5. A number of deformations consequent to the same extrinsic cause are referred to in this text as deformation sequences.

Uterine constraint tends also to reduce the rate of fetal growth and is one cause of prenatal growth deficiency. Such newborn babies frequently show deformational evidence of uterine constraint other than growth deficiency alone.

Any situation that tends to overdistend the uterus may be associated with early onset of labor, with prematurity. This is a major concern for twins who simply distend the uterus prematurely and for the woman with a bicornuate uterus of the type that tends to become overdistended before term.

If the diagnosis is not clear at the time of birth the early postnatal course may provide valuable clues as to whether the deformations noted at birth are extrinsic in causation. The otherwise normal infant who has been constrained in late fetal life tends to show progressive improvement in growth and form after being released from the deforming situation at birth. If growth has been slowed by constraint in late fetal life, the infant tends to show catch-up growth toward his or her genetic potential in early infancy, usually within the first two months. If growth of particular parts has been restrained, they tend to show catch-up growth toward normal form. This was dramatically shown to be true of nasal growth in an example of prolonged face

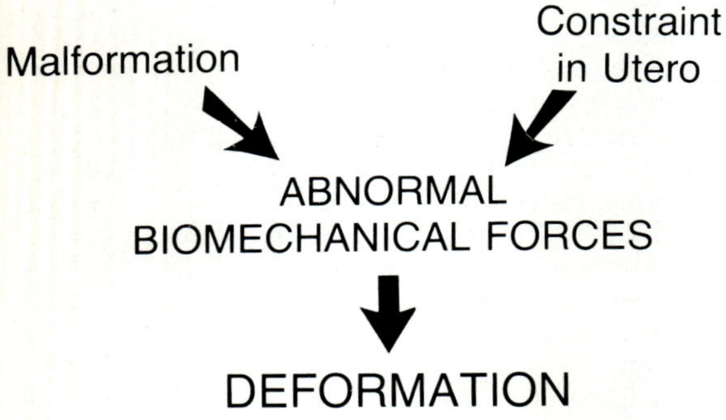

Figure 3–2. Unusual mechanical forces resulting in deformation may be the consequence of extrinsic constraint of a normal fetus or they may be the result of an intrinsic malformation of the fetus.

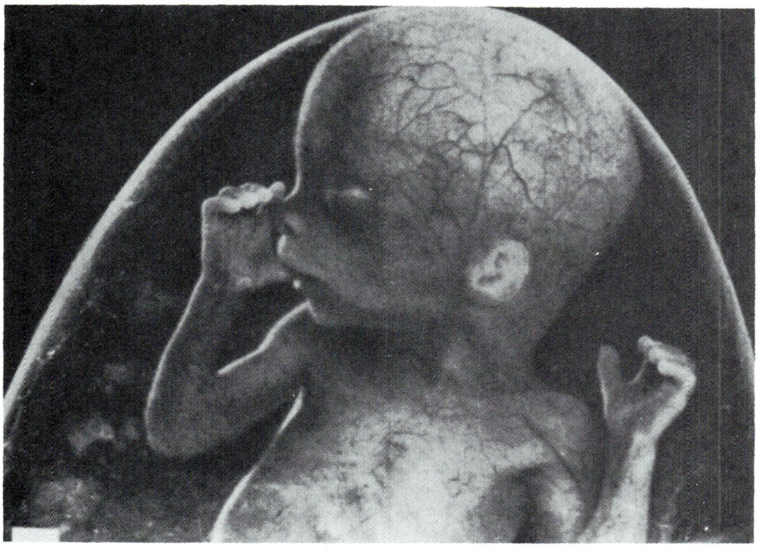

Figure 3–3. Twenty-eight week fetus with sufficient amniotic fluid such that there is no mechanical limitation to growth and morphogenesis.

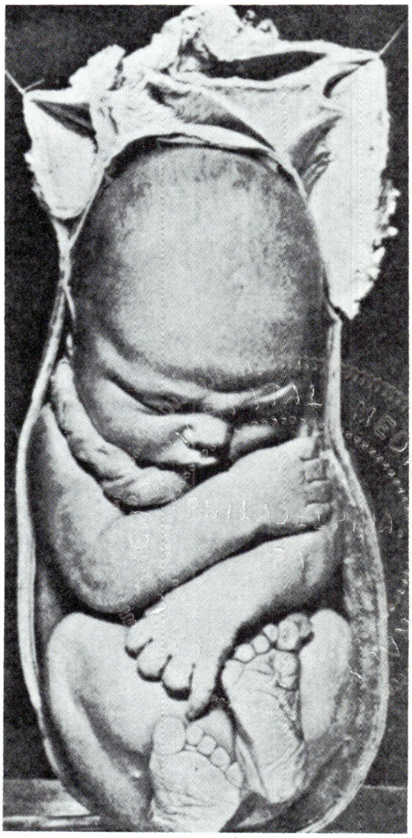

Figure 3–4. Term fetus of a primigravida in position to be born illustrating the uterine constraint which is a frequent feature in late fetal life. (The mother was killed in an auto accident and the fetus was dead on arrival at the hospital.) (From Peter Dunn, M.D., Southmead Hospital, Bristol, England.)

DEFORMITIES	compressed face	deformed head	mandibular asymmetry	torticollis	scoliosis	deformed hip	deformed foot
compressed face		+	++	+	++	++	++
deformed head	+		++	++	++	++	–
mandibular asymmetry	++	++		++	–	++	++
torticollis	+	++	++		++	–	++
scoliosis	++	++	–	++		++	+
deformed hips	++	++	++	–	++		++
deformed foot	++	–	++	++	+	++	

– not signif; + = $p<0.05$; ++ = $p<0.001$

Figure 3–5. The non-random clinical association between deformations. (Adapted from Dunn, P.M.: Proc. R. Soc. Med. *65*:735, 1972).

presentation. Joints that have been externally constrained tend to show progressive increase in their range of mobility after birth.

If there is a lack of catch-up growth and/or return toward normal form after birth, then a further evaluation may be indicated to search for a more intrinsic problem within the patient that might be responsible for the deformation(s).

HISTORICAL PERSPECTIVE

During recent times there has been less recognition of mechanical constraint factors as a cause for problems of prenatal morphogenesis than was true during some periods in past history. As far back as Hippocrates it was noted that uterine constraint could cause fetal deformation.[1] Aristotle carried out experiments which showed that crowding of chick development caused limb deformation.[5] However, there was little written about constraint deformations from then until the Renaissance era. In 1573, Ambroise Paré of France wrote that "narrowness of the uterus produces monsters by the same manner that the Dame of Paris carried the little dogs in a small basket to the end that they didn't grow." A little over a half century ago the text on *Diseases of the Newborn* by von Reuss[6] contained an entire chapter on postural deformations, whereas present day texts about the newborn have scanty coverage of this subject. One reason for the limited recognition of the more common mechanical factors in morphogenesis during the recent era may be the relative preoccupation with biochemical and physiological factors in morphogenesis. Though the latter are of obvious importance, so are the mechanical factors. This understanding is certainly important for the clinician dealing with problems of morphogenesis.

A number of investigators have made major contributions to our knowledge and understanding of extrinsic deformation during this century. A few brief summations and quotations from representative individuals will serve to emphasize some of their important observations and interpretations.

Thompson:[7] "We are ruled by gravity." "There is freedom of movement in the plane perpendicular to gravitational force." "Gravity affects stature and leads to sagging of tissues and drooping of the mouth."

von Reuss:[6] This early Viennese neonatologist made the following statement about contractural deformities: ". . .the deformities occur probably most frequently from pressure on the part by the uterine wall; sometimes marks of pressure may be observed on the skin."

Chapple and Davidson:[8] Chapple and Davidson noted that the "position of comfort" of the deformed infant soon after birth tends to be that which had existed in utero. Repositioning the baby into the "position of comfort" may allow the clinician to more readily deduce the causative compressive factors which resulted in the deformation.

Browne:[9-11] Denis Browne, who was an orthopedist at Great Ormond Street Children's Hospital in London, recognized that deformed infants were often the product of an "uncomfortable" pregnancy, implying uterine constraint. He emphasized the need for controlled forces, utilizing functional growth, in the correction of such deformations.

Dunn:[1,2] Peter Dunn, a pediatrician and neonatologist in Bristol, England, who has been responsible for resurrection and extension of knowledge about extrinsic deformation, states that "intra-uterine forces capable of moulding the fetus increase throughout pregnancy as the infant grows, the mother's uterus and abdominal wall are stretched, and the volume of amniotic fluid diminishes. At the same time the ability of the infant to resist deformation also increases as the rate of fetal growth slows, the skeleton ossifies, and leg movements become more powerful. All these factors are, of course, themselves directly or indirectly under the influence of heredity and are involved in a dynamic interplay throughout fetal life. Nature plays her hand to the limit. The price paid for a larger and more mature infant at birth, better able to withstand the stresses of extrauterine life, is a 2 per cent incidence of deformities."

FACTORS THAT ENHANCE FETAL CONSTRAINT IN UTERO

Table 3–1 summarizes some of the factors that increase the likelihood of fetal constraint in utero and these are presented in more detail below.

Table 3–1. Factors That Increase the Likelihood of Fetal Constraint in Utero

MATERNAL	Primigravida Small maternal size Small uterus Uterine malformation Uterine fibromata Small maternal pelvis
FETAL	Early pelvic engagement of the fetal head Unusual fetal position Oligohydramnios Large fetus, rapid growth Multiple fetuses

Primigravida

The first fetus may experience more constraint than later offspring because he or she is the first to distend the uterus and the mother's abdominal wall. As a consequence, most constraint types of deformations are more common in infants of primigravidas than in infants of multigravidas. Figure 3–6 shows the form of the uterus and surrounding region in a primigravida and in a multigravida, emphasizing the differences in shape and size of the tissues around the fetus. This greater magnitude of late fetal constraint in the primigravida is considered a major reason why the first born is normally smaller at birth than later born offspring. Though the first born tends to be 200 to 300 gm smaller than later offspring at birth, they are of comparable size by one year of age.[12] Thus the mild late fetal growth deficiency in the offspring of a primigravida is transient and they tend to rapidly "catch up" to their genetic pace of growth postnatally. Usually this catch-up is achieved within the first few months after birth. The first born is also more likely to become constrained in an unusual position, such as the breech presentation, and to have consequent deformations relating to such a position.

Small Mother

The smaller the mother in relation to fetal size, the greater is the liability of deforming uterine constraint in late fetal life. Thus most deformations are more common for the small woman than for the larger woman. The impact is readily evident in terms of birth size. Maternal size has a much greater impact on birth size than does paternal size. However, by one year of age the length of the infant relates equally to maternal and paternal stature.[12] Much of this maternal impact on birth size appears to relate to the transient effect of the smaller mother in restraining late fetal growth via uterine constraint. Postnatally the infant moves into his or her own genetic pace of growth, which is usually evident by one year of age. The effect of maternal size on prenatal growth is illustrated in Figures 3–7 and 3–8.

Uterine Malformation

Limitation in the capacity of the uterus to accommodate a fetus may result in early miscarriage, stillbirth, prematurity, and/or an offspring who survives to be born with sufficient constraint to give rise to deformation(s). Such reproductive problems are particularly likely to occur with uterine malformations such as a bicornuate or unicornuate uterus.[13] It is estimated that about 1 to 2 per cent of women have a uterine malformation. The likelihood of a deformation problem in

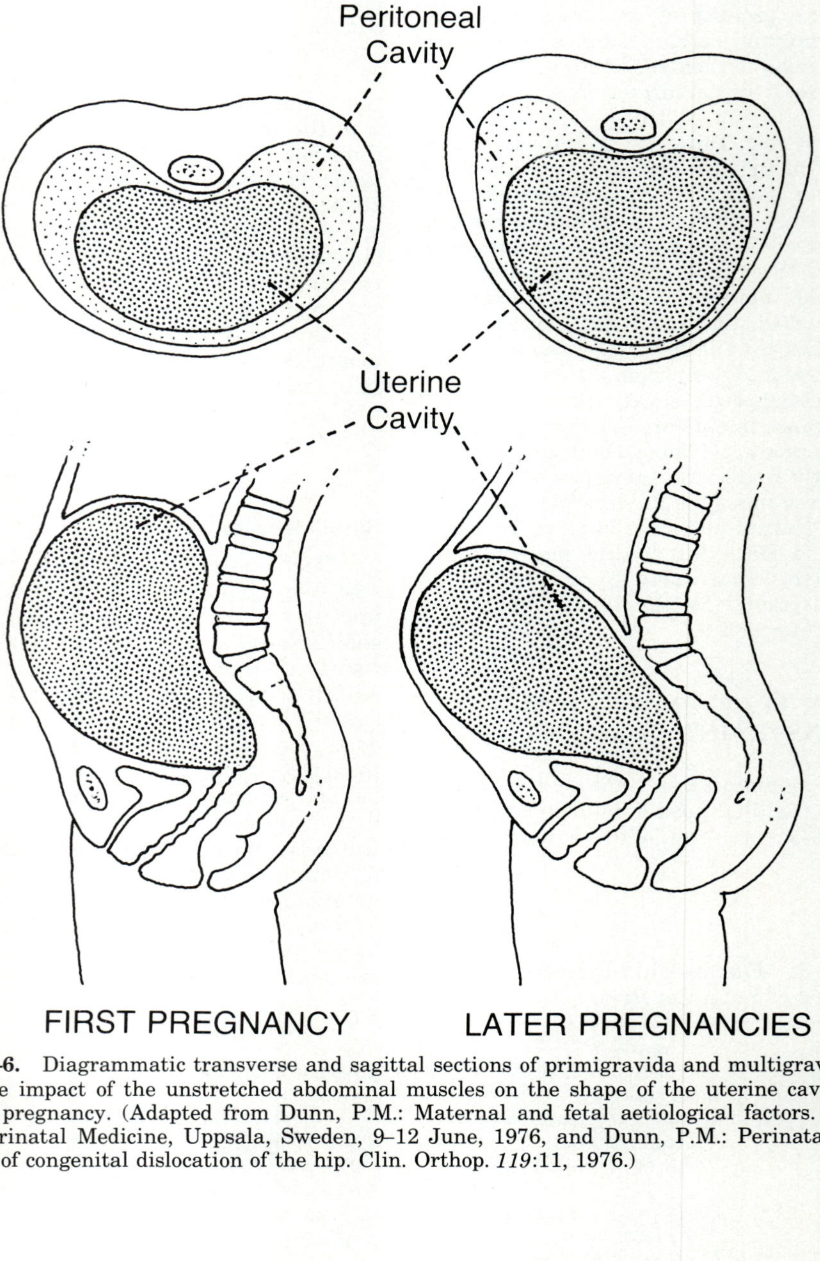

Figure 3–6. Diagrammatic transverse and sagittal sections of primigravida and multigravida abdomens to illustrate the impact of the unstretched abdominal muscles on the shape of the uterine cavity during the later weeks of pregnancy. (Adapted from Dunn, P.M.: Maternal and fetal aetiological factors. 5th European Congress of Perinatal Medicine, Uppsala, Sweden, 9–12 June, 1976, and Dunn, P.M.: Perinatal observations on the etiology of congenital dislocation of the hip. Clin. Orthop. *119*:11, 1976.)

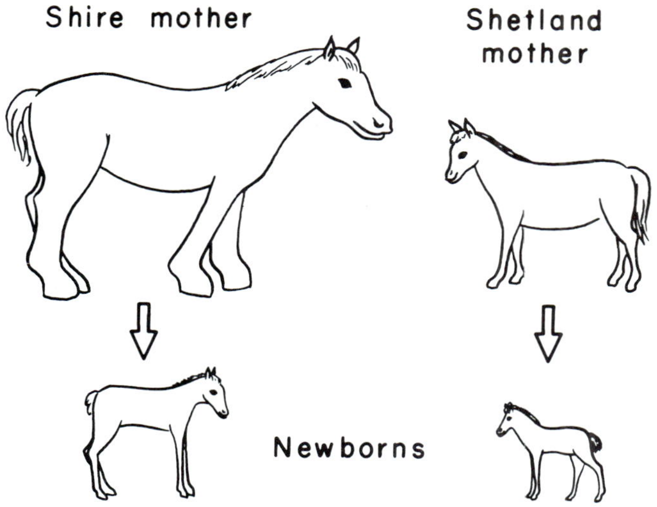

Figure 3–7. Influence of maternal size on the size of the offspring at birth is dramatically illustrated by the cross between a shire horse and a Shetland pony. Though the genetic situation is the same, the foal of the small mother is much smaller than that of the large mother, presumably because of the smaller space within which to rear the fetus. (Adapted from Hammond, J.: Growth in size and body proportions in farm animals. In Zarrow, M.X.: Growth in Living Systems. New York, Basic Books Inc. 1961, p. 321.)

the fetus reared in a bicornuate uterus has been crudely estimated to be about 30 per cent.[13] The recognition that a malformation of the uterus has caused a fetal problem may lead to corrective surgery of the uterus, thus providing a better opportunity for the next fetus to grow without as much constraint.

Uterine Fibromata

A large fibroid of the uterus may limit intrauterine space and therefore have gestational impact similar to that of a bicornuate uterus. The possibility of surgical removal of the tumor, allowing for better fetal space, merits consideration in such cases. Fortunately most uterine fibromata develop either late in reproductive life or after reproduction and are an infrequent cause of fetal deformation. However, a small fibroma may grow rapidly during gestation under the high level estrogen effects.

Small Maternal Pelvis

Vaginal delivery through a small pelvic outlet in relationship to the size of the fetus may result in appreciable molding of the craniofacies. This is usually quite transient. However, if there has been prolonged engagement of the fetal head into a small pelvis the degree of molding can be severe and there may be a rather slow resolution toward normal form postnatally.

Early Pelvic Engagement of the Fetal Head

Early descent of the fetal head into the maternal pelvis is often accompanied by maternal symptoms of pelvic pressure and discomfort that sometimes include pains radiating down the legs while walking. It is very unusual for the fetal head to descend more than six weeks before term, and it seldom does so more than one month

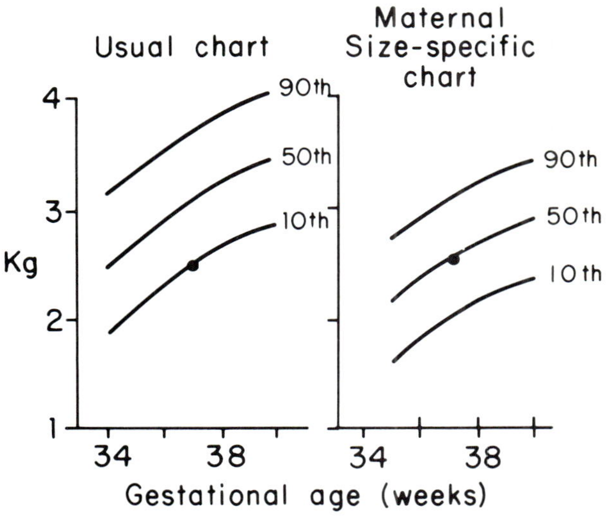

Figure 3–8. The weight of a 2.3 kg newborn baby born to a small mother with a weight of 40 kg and height of 150 cm, plotted on a usual grid (left) and on one that is specific for maternal size (right). (Adapted from Winick, M.: Biologic correlations. Am. J. Dis. Child. *120*:416, 1970. Standards to the right are from Thomson, A. M., et al.: The assessment of fetal growth. J. Obstet. Gynec. Brit. Comm. *75*:903, 1968.)

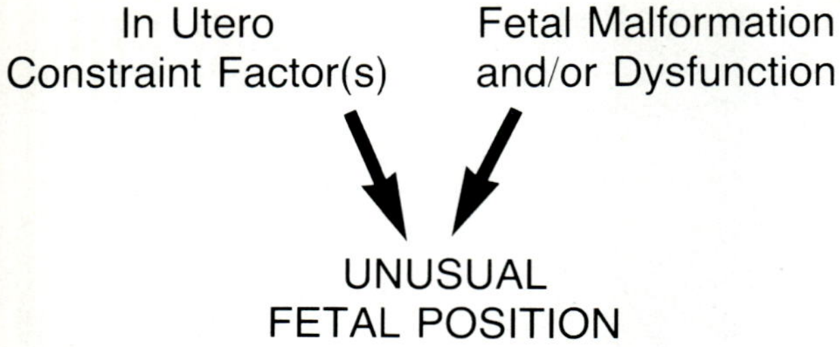

Figure 3–9. Unusual fetal position in utero may be the result of constraint factors to a normal fetus, or it may be the consequence of a primary fetal malformation and/or dysfunction.

prior to delivery. Early fetal head descent is more common in the primigravida. When the symptoms are severe, it may be difficult for the mother to walk during the later period of gestation. The fetal consequences are predominantly craniofacial deformation. One potential result is vertex craniotabes,[4] secondary to prolonged compression of the top of the calvarium, resulting in poorly mineralized, malleable bone in the region of compression. Another potential consequence is constraint of fetal head growth in one dimension, resulting in a lack of growth stretch across one or more of the sutures. If there is a lack of growth stretch across a given suture, then that suture is more liable to become ossified and result in a craniosynostosis problem.[15]

Fetal Position

Prior to 36 to 37 weeks from conception, when the fetus usually has adequate room for movement in its aquatic environment, it is not unusual for the fetus to be in varying positions, including breech presentation. As the fetus becomes more crowded, he or she will tend to shift into the vertex presentation position, there being more room in the fundal portion of the uterus for the bulkier legs.

Unusual late fetal position in utero may result from a number of factors, as summarized in Figures 3–9 and 3–10. This may be the consequence of a primary fetal neuromuscular problem, which limited the ability of the fetus to move in utero, and/or of a malformation that altered the form or function of the fetus. The more common reason for aberrant fetal position is in-utero constraint which has limited the capacity of the fetus to move into the vertex presentation. Abnormal fetal position during late fetal life may result in unusual constraint forces on fetal morphogenesis. Examples, which are set forth in Chapter Two, include breech presentation, face presentation, brow presentation, and transverse lie. Breech presentation, though occurring only in about 4 per cent of pregnancies, is associated with about 32 per cent of all extrinsic deformations.[16]

Large Fetus, Rapid Growth

The fetus manifests a rapid rate of growth. For example, it doubles in weight during the six week period from 28 to 34 weeks in utero. The faster the growth rate and the larger the fetus, the greater is the liability toward external constraint types of deformation. The male is normally larger and grows more rapidly in late fetal life than does the female. Therefore, most extrinsic deformations are more common in the male than in the female, except for dislocation of the hip and other deformations that appear to relate to greater connective tissue laxity in females.

Multiple Fetuses

Multiple fetuses fill out the uterine cavity sooner than average. The average uterus is capable of handling about 4 kg of fetal mass. For twins this combined size is usually achieved by

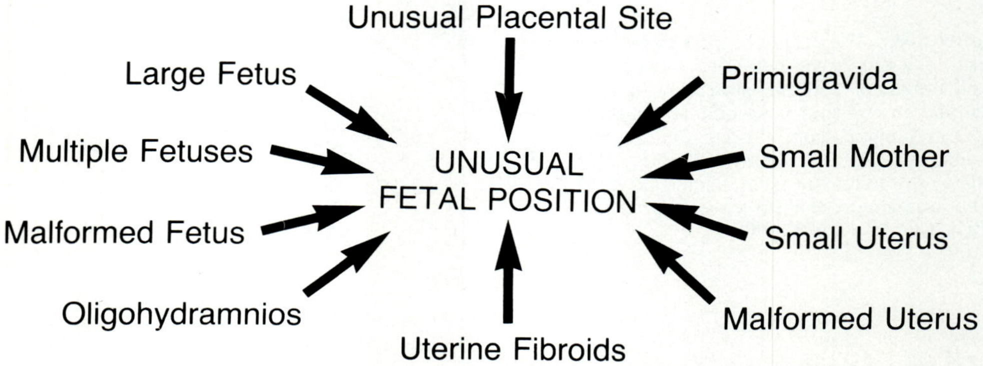

Figure 3–10. Maternal and fetal factors that can result in unusual position of the fetus in utero.

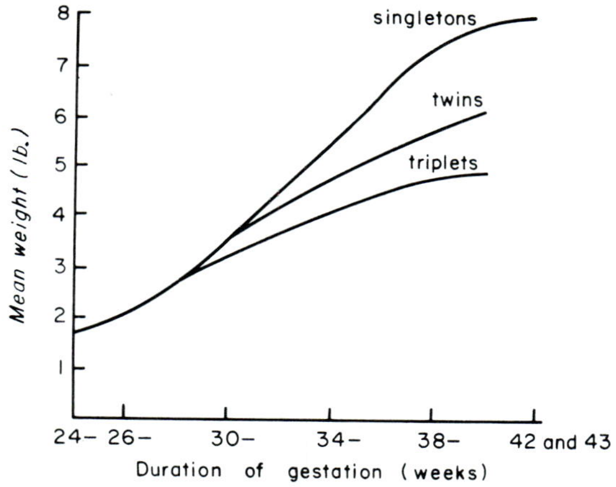

Figure 3–11. The mean fetal weights of singletons as compared to twins and triplets. While the initial growth rate is the same, the combined size of twins or triplets leads to earlier uterine constraint and late fetal slowing of growth. (Adapted from Bulmer, M.G.: The Biology of Twinning in Man. Oxford, Clarendon Press, 1970.)

about the thirty-fourth week of gestation; thereafter there tends to be a slowing in growth as the uterine cavity becomes filled,[11] as is shown in Figure 3–11. Other deformations besides transient growth deficiency also tend to be more common in twins, especially malpositioning of feet and molding of the craniofacies. This is one reason why monozygotic twins may not appear to be identical at the time of birth. One of the twins may have been constrained in a different manner and to a different degree than the other twin. Some of this may relate to aberrant fetal positioning, especially the breech presentation in one of the twins.

Oligohydramnios

A deficit of amniotic fluid in late fetal life may be due to a variety of causes, such as early rupture of the amnion with chronic leakage of amniotic fluid, lack of urine flow into the amniotic space, or maternal hypertension. However, regardless of the cause, a lack of amniotic fluid tends to give rise to an unusual degree of uterine constraint, which affects fetal growth, including thoracic and lung growth, and may also cause a number of craniofacial and limb deformations.[17] The consequences are referred to as the *oligohydramnios sequence.* The impact of oligohydramnios versus polyhydramnios on birth size is shown in Figure 3–12.

PROGNOSIS, MANAGEMENT, AND COUNSEL

When a deformation is due to external constraint in late fetal life in an otherwise normal individual, the prognosis for a return to normal form is usually excellent. The management of extrinsic deformations may vary with the cause. Sometimes it is worthwhile to simply observe the spontaneous changes for several days to several weeks after birth before making a decision as to whether any therapy is indicated. The mode of treatment may simply utilize corrective mechanical forces similar to those that gave rise to the deformation in striving to *force* the deformed tissues into a more normal form. When possible, this mechanical therapy should take advantage of normal growth. However, there should be caution in attempting to treat a deformation with a mode of management that may produce additional deformations.

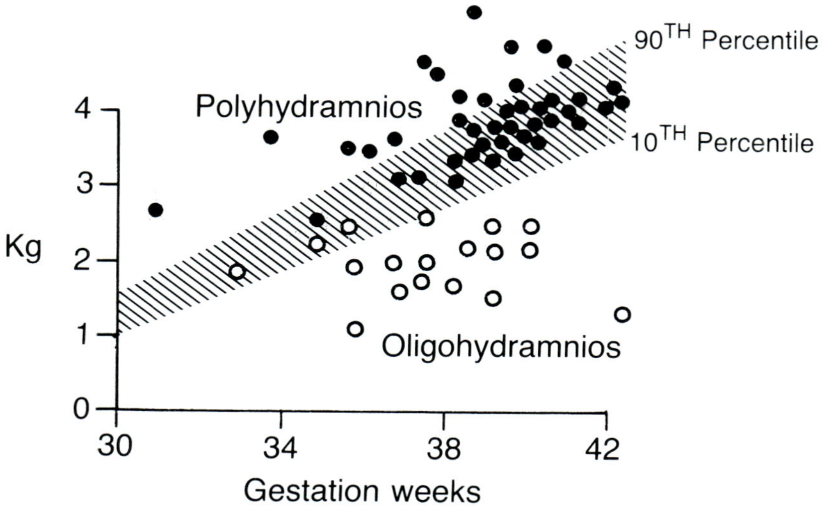

Figure 3–12. Impact on birth weight in kilograms of oligohydramnios due to renal insufficiency (open dots) versus polyhydramnios (solid dots). (Adapted from Dunn, P.M.: Growth retardation of infants with congenital postural deformities. Acta. Med. Auxol. 7:63, 1975.)

The actual modes of management for reforming constraint deformations may vary appreciably and yet accomplish the same purpose. Simple manual manipulation with molding and stretching toward normal form may be all that is needed. This is a common and ancient practice in India, where "massage women" are employed to mold and shape the baby. They come to the home daily for two to three months, or as long as indicated. By massage with oil and stretching, they form the baby into a normal shape and remove any extrinsic deformations that may have been present at birth. In a similar fashion, parents can be instructed to accomplish such molding or stretching at home. More consistent forces may be applied to foot deformities by frequent adhesive taping, with gradual improvement in the form. When such benign measures do not result in improvement, more rigorous means of molding and stretching, such as casting of the limbs or helmet molding of the head, may be utilized. When a joint is seriously dislocated or malpositioned and conservative measures have not been successful in accomplishing a repositioning to normal form, surgical intervention may be indicated. Ideally, this should be done as soon as it is established that conservative measures are not working. The tendency is toward earlier surgery for such defects. This is especially important for severe equinovarus deformity in which the calcaneus and talus are at least partially dislocated. Proper bony alignment is necessary to foster normal subsequent joint development.

The counsel given to parents of a baby with an extrinsic deformation problem can usually be quite favorable. With rare exception the parents may be counseled in the following manner: "I believe your baby is normal. He (or she) became crowded in the uterus before birth and this resulted in the somewhat unusual features at birth. Having been released from this constraint, the baby's features will return toward normal with no after effects. It is for this reason that I say your baby is normal." Any treatment that is merited is then explained to the parents, as is the recurrence risk. The recurrence risk depends on the cause of the extrinsic deformation. For most deformations the recurrence risk is low. However, it may be quite high if the cause is a persisting one, such as a uterine malformation.

Obviously, it is important to distinguish between an extrinsic deformation and an intrinsic deformation problem secondary to a malformation, since this distinction has major impact on the prognosis and management of the child and on the recurrence risk for the parents.

PREVENTION

At first thought, the prevention of extrinsic deformation seems an unlikely possibility. However, there already exist several examples of preventive measures and more may be developed in the future. Surgical repair of a malformed uterus that has been shown to cause serious problems for fetal survival and deformation[13] may be followed by a greatly improved prognosis for a normal offspring. A more controversial preventive measure is external version of the fetus who is in an aberrant position in utero. This is usually accomplished (by those rare physicians who practice external version) by 34 to 35 weeks from conception. After 35 weeks of gestation it is more difficult to accomplish external version of the fetus into the vertex presentation. The most common potential indication for external version is breech presentation. In the experience of one obstetrician who routinely practices external version for malposition in utero,[18] there has been a 0.54 per cent incidence of breech presentation at term. This is much less than the 3.5 per cent general frequency of breech presentation at term when external version has not been utilized. Since breech presentation has been considered responsible for almost one third of the extrinsic deformations and one half of the cases of dislocation of the hip in Dunn's series of some 6000 babies,[16] any reduction in the frequency of breech presentation at term might have quite an impact on the frequency of deformations, especially dislocation of the hip. However, there are risks involved in the procedure of external version, and it is a technique that is not routinely taught. Dr. Brooks Ranney of Yankton, South Dakota, has performed external version on about 10 per cent of 7000 pregnant women. He utilizes external version as early as the twenty-eighth week of gestation, but more commonly at 30 to 34 weeks. Approximately 20 to 30 per cent of the fetuses revert, and external version is again carried out, up to as many as eight times. The contraindications to external version include multiple pregnancy, placenta previa, unicornuate uterus, and gross obesity. Anesthesia is never used. The version is accomplished by gentle maneuvering while monitoring the fetal heart. Dr. Ranney has not had any fatality related to the procedure. Hopefully, more studies will be done to better determine whether the value of external version of the malpositioned fetus in utero is greater than the harm that may be done by the procedure. The question has not been fully resolved at this time, although the majority of obstetricians do not utilize external version in practice.

Prevention of the serious problems that are secondary to constraint deformation merits comment. One example is the scaphocephalic head with prominent occiput that may develop following prolonged breech presentation in late fetal life.[19] This so-called breech head is itself usually a benign deformation that tends to resolve postnatally. However, the contour of this head can pose serious problems during vaginal delivery, because it tends to become arrested during the second stage of labor. This complication increases the liability for brachial plexus tears and cord trauma with neurological residua during a vaginal delivery. Detection of the "breech head" by ultrasonography or radiography may warrant cesarean section delivery of such a fetus in breech presentation. Thus, prenatal detection of such a deformation may influence management toward prevention of serious high-risk vaginal birth trauma.

INTERACTIONS BETWEEN EXTRINSIC AND INTRINSIC FACTORS YIELDING DEFORMATION

A given deformation might relate to both extrinsic and intrinsic factors, representing an interaction between the two. One example is dislocation of the hip (Fig. 3–13). According to the author's judgment, most instances of dislocation of the hip are secondary to external constraint, which forces the hip out of its socket by stretching the joint capsule and the ligamentum teres. Dislocation of the hip is hypothesized to be more common in the female because the female fetus has more laxity of connective tissue than the male. This is presumed to be the consequence of a lack of testosterone in the female fetus, the assumption being that the testosterone yields tougher connective tissue in the male fetus.[20] Dislocation of the hip may also result from an intrinsic abnormality in the fetus having unduly lax connective tissue.[21] This can usually be discerned clinically by noting laxity in other joints in a patient with dislocation of the hip.

Another example of the interaction between intrinsic and extrinsic factors in creating a deformation is the fetus who has an intrinsic problem, such as a neuromuscular abnormality, that limits the ability of the fetus to turn into the vertex position before birth. Such a fetus is more likely to be caught in the breech position and to be born with such problems as "breech head," dislocation of the hip, and other deformities that are more likely to occur to the fetus who is in the breech position.

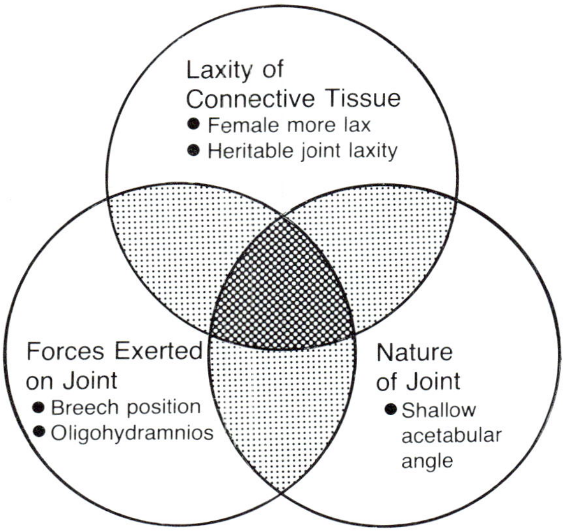

Figure 3–13. Interacting factors may relate to the liability to develop a deformation such as dislocation of the hip.

INTRINSIC CAUSATION OF DEFORMATION

The cause of a given deformation may be altered mechanical forces as the consequence of a more *primary* problem within the fetus, such as a malformation. Although these intrinsic deformations are not the main subject of this book, it is important to be aware of them in the differential diagnosis of extrinsic deformations. Some of these deformations may be caused by either extrinsic factors or intrinsic ones. For example, the same type of malposition of the foot may be the consequence of external constraint of the foot, of neurological deficit, or of a muscle disorder. The judgment of the clinician is required in order to determine the *primary* causation for the deformation. The overall diagnosis, prognosis, and recurrence risk counsel for the child with a malpositioned foot may differ widely if the deformation is secondary to uterine constraint rather than due to a primary neuromuscular problem.

There are several types of intrinsic fetal problems that may result in altered mechanics and thereby give rise to deformation of otherwise normal tissues. Examples include neuromuscular disorders, aberrant growth of a tissue, and obstruction of a hollow viscus. Examples of each are set forth below:

Neuromuscular Problems

A deficit of neuromuscular function may result in multiple deformations. When the primary problem is neural, there may be a secondary loss of muscle mass. As a consequence of diminished movement, there may be joint fixations. Also, with a lack of stress the bone grows more slowly in breadth, tending to become more slender. Sites of muscle attachment to bone, which are normally prominent, may be less prominent or even lacking as a result of the neuromuscular deficiency.

Excessive neuromuscular function, such as spasticity, may give rise to unusual magnitude and direction of muscle forces with consequent mechanical effects on morphogenesis.

Localized Growth Deficiency

Localized growth deficiency of one tissue may give rise to subsequent deformational problems in adjacent tissues. One such example is localized growth deficiency of the mandible. If this occurs in early morphogenesis it tends to place the tongue in a posterior location in the oropharynx. If this happens before 9 to 10 weeks of fetal life, prior to the closure of the palatal shelves, the tongue may obstruct full palatal shelf closure, yielding a U-shaped palatal defect.[22] Once the baby is born there may be upper airway obstruction secondary to the retroplaced tongue. The combined findings are referred to as the Robin malformation sequence, previously referred to as the Pierre Robin syndrome. Beyond the initiating malformation of a small mandible, the remaining features are deformations, the consequences of altered biomechanics engendered by the small mandible.

Localized Overgrowth

A localized overgrowth may cause mechanical problems in the adjacent region. This is obvious with most tumors. One example is a nasopharyngeal teratoma, which can obstruct palatine closure and partially occlude the upper airway, yielding deformational features similar to those noted for the Robin sequence.

Obstruction of a Hollow Viscus

Obstruction of a hollow organ will result in altered mechanics with increased pressures and deformations of the expanded tissue as well as distortion of tissues that surround the enlarging hollow structure. Examples include obstructive hydrocephalus, intestinal obstruction, and obstruction in the urogenital system. One dramatic illustration is the urethral obstruction sequence as shown in Figure 3–14, which has been more commonly termed the "prune belly syndrome."[23] Most commonly the primary malformation is an obstruction in the development of the penile urethra. This results in massive enlargement of the bladder and the ureters. The back pressure adversely affects renal morphogenesis. The enlarging bladder distends the abdomen, causing diminished abdominal musculature. It also prevents full rotation of the gut, resulting in malrotation, and it obstructs full descent of the testes. The horrendous compressive effects of the distended bladder are usually lethal in early fetal life unless the bladder "blows out," either by rupturing an obstructing urethral valve or by way of the urachus, which tends to remain patent as a consequence of the pressure, or by rupture of the bladder or ureter. Once the bladder is decom-

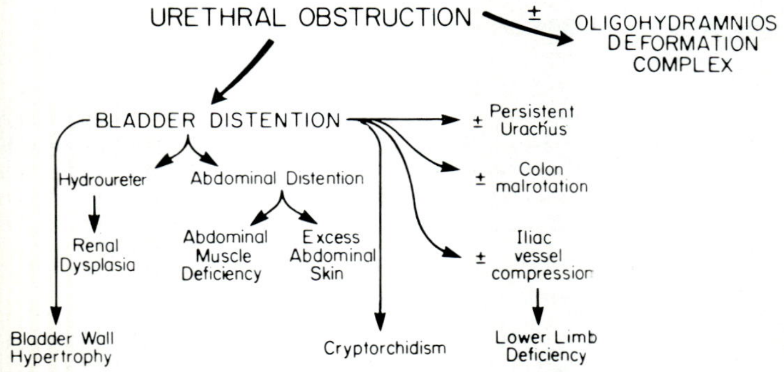

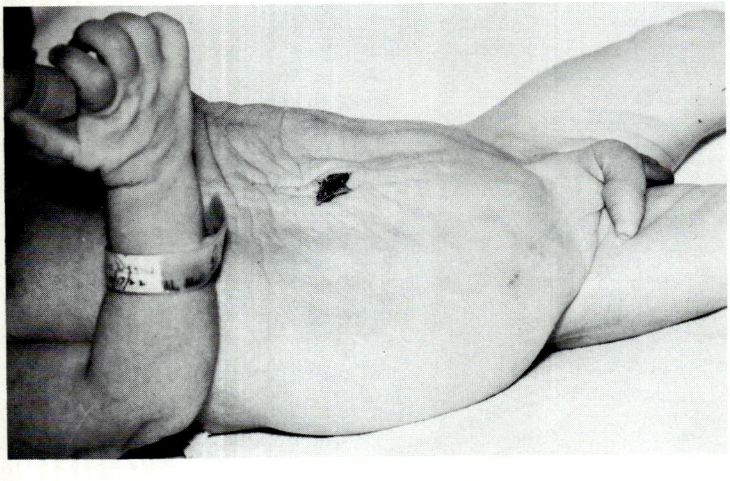

Figure 3–14. The development of the urethral obstruction sequence. The initiating malformation is most commonly urethral obstruction. All the other features are deformations due to the back pressure in the urinary system. In order to survive to a term birth the distended bladder must decompress, thus yielding the "prune belly" abdomen as shown below. (Top from Pagon, R.A., Smith, D.W., and Shepard, T.H.: J. Pediatr. *96*:900, 1979.)

pressed, the fetus is left with a lax abdomen with redundant folds of excess skin, the so-called "prune belly." Thus all these deformations are secondary to one primary intrinsic malformation, early urethral obstruction. Similar distention and muscular thinning of the abdomen can be seen with congenital ascites, which may result from a variety of causes.

The heart is a hollow viscus in which, as it develops, alterations in the direction or magnitude of blood flow, such as may be caused by partial obstructions, may give rise to secondary deformation in both form and size.

REFERENCES

1. Dunn, P.M.: The influence of the intrauterine environment in the causation of congenital postural deformities, with special reference to congenital dislocation of the hip. (Thesis for M.D. degree.) University of Cambridge, 1969.
2. Dunn, P.M.: Congenital postural deformities. Br. Med. Bull. *32*:71, 1976.
3. Harrison, R.G., and Malpas, P.: The volume of human amniotic fluid. J. Obstet. Gynaec. Brit. Emp. *60*:632, 1953.
4. Nishimura, H., *In* Fraser, F.C., and McKusick, V.A. (eds.): Congenital Malformations. (International Congress Series, no. 204.) Amsterdam, Excerpta Medica, 1970, p. 275.
5. Tarruffi, C.: Storia della teratologia. (History of teratology.) Bologna, Regia Tipografia, 1881.
6. von Reuss, A.R.: The Diseases of the Newborn. New York, William Wood and Co., 1921.
7. Thompson, d'A.W.: On Growth and Form. A New Edition. Cambridge, The University Press, 1942.
8. Chapple, C.C., and Davidson, D.T.: A study of the relationship between fetal position and certain congenital deformities. J. Pediatr. *18*:483, 1941.
9. Browne, D.: Talipes equino-varus. Lancet *2*:969, 1934.
10. Browne, D.: Congenital deformities of mechanical origin. Proc. Roy. Soc. Med. *29*:1409, 1935–36.
11. Browne, D.: Congenital deformities of mechanical origin. Arch. Dis. Child. *30*:37, 1955.
12. Smith, D.W.: Growth and Its Disorders. W.B. Saunders Co., Philadelphia, 1975.
13. Miller, M.E., Dunn, P.M., and Smith, D.W.: Uterine malformation and fetal deformation. J. Pediatr. *94*:387, 1979.
14. Graham, J.M., and Smith, D.W.: Parietal craniotabes in the neonate: Its origin and relevance. J. Pediatr. *95*:114, 1979.
15. Graham, J.M., deSaxe, M., and Smith, D.W.: Sagittal craniostenosis: Fetal head constraint as one possible cause. J. Pediatr. *95*:747, 1979.
16. Dunn, P.M.: Breech presentation. Maternal and fetal aetiological factors. 5th European Congress of Perinatal Medicine, Uppsala, Sweden, 1976, p. 76.
17. Thomas, I.T. and Smith, D.W.: Oligohydramnios, cause of the nonrenal features of Potter's syndrome, including pulmonary hypoplasia. J. Pediatr. *84*:811, 1974.
18. Ranney, B.: The gentle art of external cephalic version. Am. J. Obstet. Gynecol. *116*:239, 1973.
19. Haberkern, C.M., Smith, D.W., and Jones, K.L.: The "breech head" and its relevance. Am. J. Dis. Child. *133*:154, 1979.
20. Arena, J.F.P., and Smith, D.W.: Sex liability to single structural defects. Am. J. Dis. Child. *132*:970, 1978.
21. Carter, C.O., and Wilkinson, J.A.: Joint and environmental factors in the etiology of dislocation of the hip. Clin. Orthop. Rel. Res. *33*:March-April, 1964.
22. Hanson, J.W., and Smith, D.W.: U-shaped palatal defect in the Robin anomalad: Developmental and clinical relevance. J. Pediatr. *87*:30, July 1975.
23. Pagon, R.A., Smith, D.W., and Shepard, T.H.: Urethral obstruction malformation complex: A cause of abdominal muscle deficiency and the "prune belly." J. Pediatr. *95*:900, 1979.

Chapter Four

MECHANICS IN MORPHOGENESIS: PRINCIPLES AND RESPONSE OF PARTICULAR TISSUES

PRINCIPLES IN BIOMECHANICS

Rather simple principles apply for the role of mechanical factors in morphogenesis. These are that the direction and magnitude of forces affect the form of the developing individual, as illustrated in Figure 4–1. Some of the factors that affect the magnitude and direction of forces are summarized in Table 4–1. One major influence on the nature and alignment of forces is *growth*. Thus, the rate and shape of growth in a particular basic tissue will determine the magnitude and direction of the forces it exerts on adjacent tissues. The plasticity of a tissue is another factor that affects its liability to be altered by mechanical forces. The tissues of the fetus are pliable and easily molded. Another major influence is tension or compression related to muscle pull, gravity, or local constraint. The orientation within many tissues is determined by such forces. For example, collagen fibers, the basic threads and fibers of connective tissue, align in the direction of stress (see Fig. 4–2). The strands are spun out by the fibroblast cells under genetic direction, but the alignment of the fibrils in the extracellular space appears to be predominantly determined by mechanical forces. If there is no consistent direction of mechanical forces, the collagen strands are haphazardly arranged. Given a sustained direction of forces they become organized and woven in relation to those forces.

The general precepts of mechanical engineering are relevant to man, as is the nomenclature (see Table 4–2).

In many tissues there is an integral interaction between growth and the forces of tension and compression. This is readily evident in the relationship between muscle usage and the size of muscle mass. The greater the forces, the larger the muscle mass tends to become. In turn, the stress of muscle tendon pull on a bone affects the growth and form of the bone. The greater the pull of a muscle on a bone, the greater is the size of the bony promontory at the site of the tension on the bone. For example, the prominent bony ridge down the center of the skull in the male gorilla shown in Figure 4–3 relates to the size of the attachment of the powerful temporalis chewing muscles. The female gorilla does not have this prominent ridge because her muscles are less powerful.

Table 4–1. Factors Affecting the Magnitude and Direction of Mechanical Forces

External resistance to growth and/or movement
Growth rate and shape of basic tissues
Forces of fluid flow (or pressure)
Plasticity of fetus
Forces of muscle pull
Forces of gravity

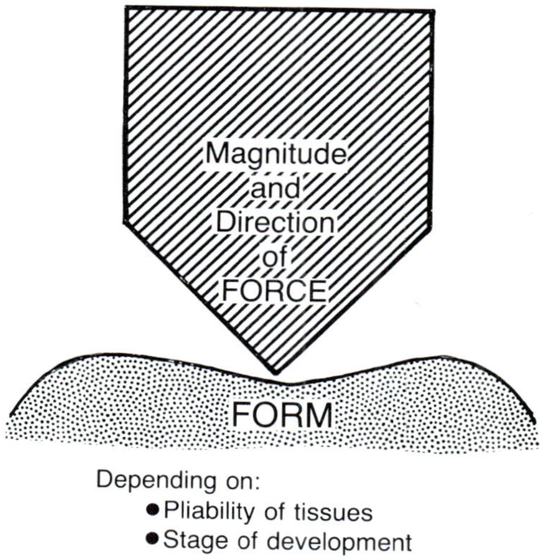

Figure 4–1. The basic principles relative to deformation are simple — the magnitude and direction of forces have their impact on form. The response of a given tissue is dependent on its pliability and stage of development.

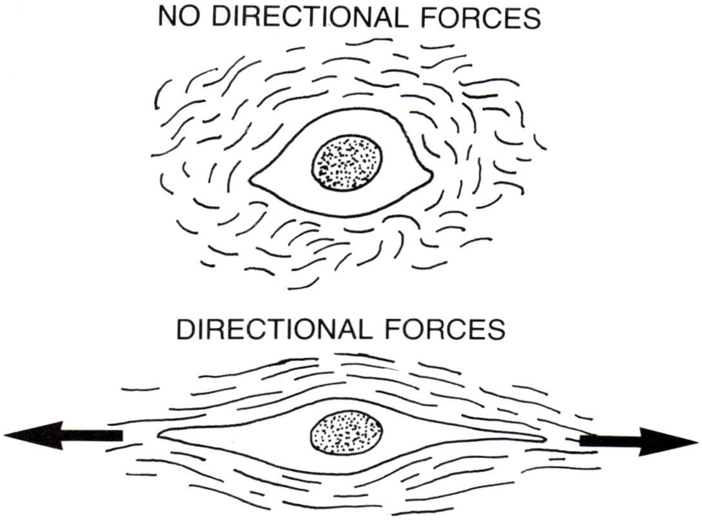

Figure 4–2. Schematic depiction of fibroblasts producing collagen fibrils. When there are no directional forces the extruded fibrils tend to be haphazardly oriented (above). When there are directional forces, the collagen fibrils align in the direction of the forces, thus affecting the form of the tissue. (From discussions with Prof. Gian Töndury, Anatomisches Institute, University of Zurich.)

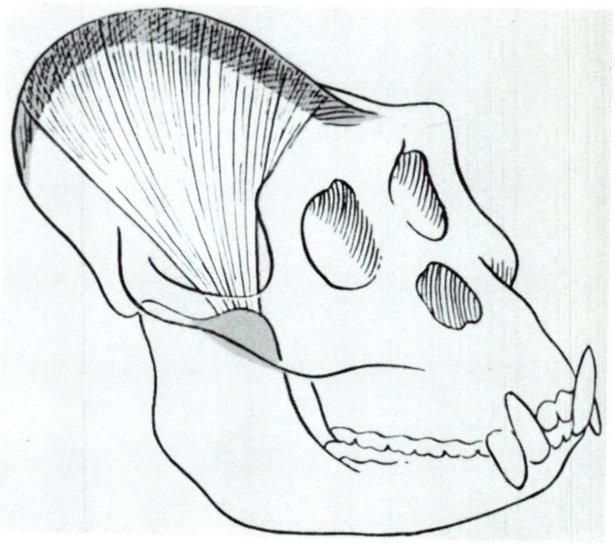

Figure 4–3. Male gorilla skull with prominent bony ridge down the center of the calvarium which is the consequence of the pull of the powerful temporalis muscles, which insert at this location.

Table 4–2. Mechanical Engineering Terms That Are Applicable to Man

Deformation	altered form due to unusual forces
Stress	intensity of force (force per unit area)
Strain	sufficient force to cause deformation
Tension	stretching forces
Compression	compressive forces
Torsion	twisting forces
Shear forces	forces contrary to the main orientation of a material or tissue

We are ruled by gravity, which has a major impact on our form. Since our relative surface area to overall volume proportion is small, we are ruled by gravitational forces acting upon weight. In contrast, gravity is relatively negligible to very small animals that have a high surface area to volume ratio. Their world is more dominated by surface forces.

Examples of the impact of mechanical forces on morphogenesis abound in nature. The magnitude and direction of growth on form is dramatically reflected in the chambered nautilus, whose shell represents the successively larger living quarters occupied by this mollusk as it outgrows and creates one new chamber after another, resulting in an equiangular logarithmic spiral shell, as shown in Figure 4–4. This also exemplifies the basic orderliness of the growth and its biomechanical consequences on the form of the organism.

Another beautiful example from nature of the impact of the size and direction of forces on form is the alignment of cellulose fibers in a tree. The reason the tree grows straight up relates to the cellulose fibers aligning in the direction of the stress force of gravity. Extrinsic forces, such as compression by snow during the winter, may deform the young tree. However, once released from such temporary constraint the sapling will again tend to grow in the direction of the force of gravity. The forces of prevailing winds may be sufficient to deform a tree. Controlled external forces may be utilized to deform a young tree into an aberrant form, a form that will be maintained after the tree is fully grown. Illustrative examples are shown in Figure 4–5.

The collagen fibrils within developing bone may be compared with the cellulose fibers of a tree. They are the basic structural elements and they align in the direction of stress in such a manner as to avoid shear forces, as previously indicated. This is dramatically evidenced in the longitudinal section of the human femur shown in Figure 4–6. The bone spicules are aligned in the direction of the stress of gravitational weight bearing and also of muscle pull. The form of the upper femur relates to the combined forces of weight bearing *plus* the pull of major muscle groups. This results in a sloping "neck" of the femur and the two large promontories of bone, the greater and lesser trochanters, in this region of the femur. The force lines that are evident in the form of such a bone may be of value to the engineer in his or her design of somewhat similar structures. D'Arcy Thompson[1] relates the story of a Zürich engineer, Professor Culmann, who became famous for his design of a mechanical crane. In the design of his crane he utilized stress forces that he observed in a longitudinal section of the human femur in 1871. When shown the section of the femur by his friend, Professor Hermann von Meyer of the Anatomy Institute of the University of Zürich, Professor Culmann exclaimed, "There is my crane!" Possibly, there should be a closer interchange between biology and engineering, since the biomechanically determined "lines of stress" are naturally evident in many living creatures. The differences in these lines of stress will vary with the function of a bone. In the wings

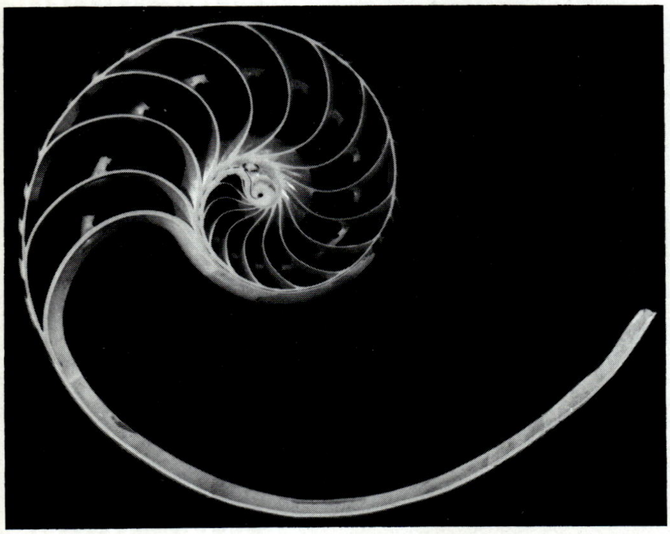

Figure 4–4. The growing nautilus mollusk outgrows one chamber after another, thus creating an equiangular logarithmic spiral shell.

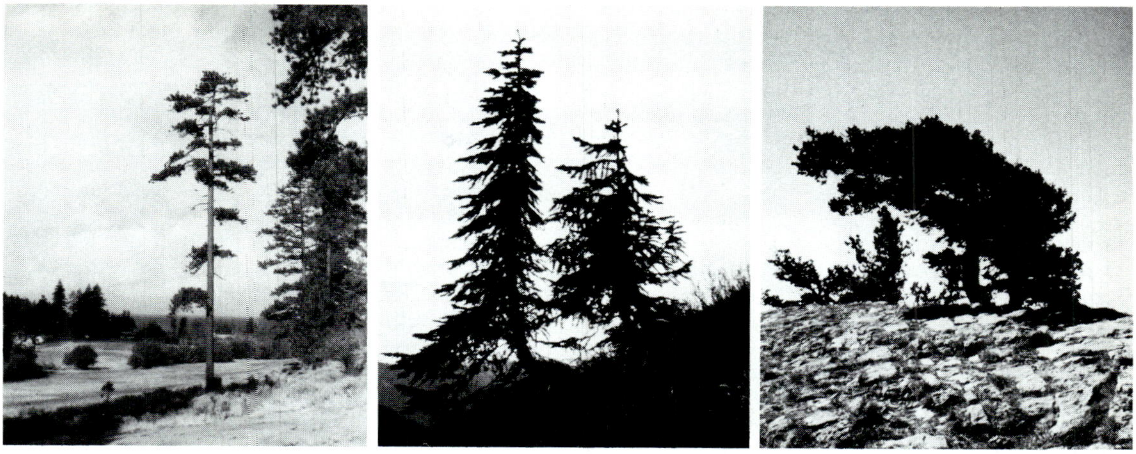

Figure 4–5. *Left,* Tree in a protected meadow location, growing straight up in relation to gravity. *Middle,* Alpine tree showing deformation of the lower trunk secondary to downward compression by the snow pack during the long winters in the early years of its growth. *Right,* Ridge-top tree showing deformation by the prevailing winds, which are from right to left.

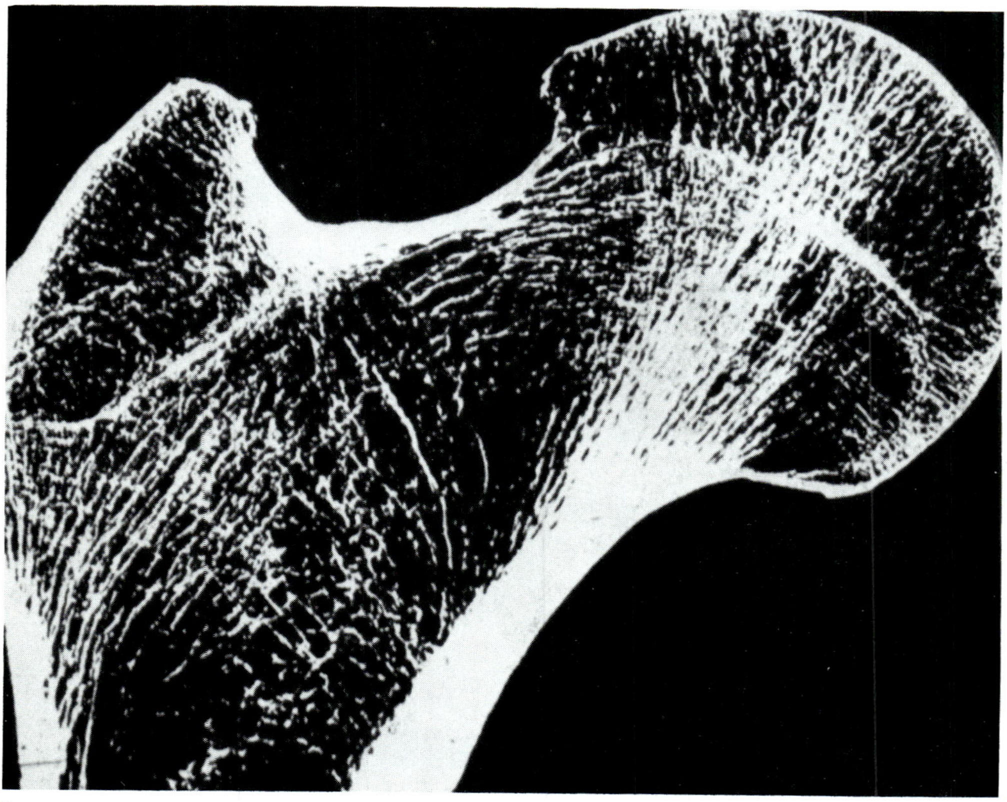

Figure 4–6. This section of the proximal human femur beautifully illustrates the relationship between function and form in the alignment of the bone spicules, which relate to the orientation of collagen fibrils. (From Thompson, d'Arcy: On Growth and Form. A New Edition. Cambridge, The University Press, 1942.)

of a soaring bird, such as the vulture, the lines of stress relate to forces above and beneath the wing. The bone form in the pneumatized bone of the vulture is aligned accordingly and appears remarkably similar to the form that engineers learned to utilize in the wing girders of early airplanes and in bridge trusses, as shown in Figure 4–7.

Mechanical forces play a major role in the form of an individual, and relate to the function of the individual. An example is the pneumatized lightweight but strong bones of the larger soaring birds. The largest soaring mammal, the extinct Pteradon shown in Figure 4–8, had a wing span of 7 meters. It apparently had pneumatized wing bones. The form and dimension of the reconstructed pteradon are considered aerodynamically ideal for the soaring function of this animal. Because its femora were delicately built and would not withstand compressive stress, it was necessary for it to hang upside down from cliffs as compensation for reduction in weight for flight. This adaptation is also true of the bat.

The evolutionary impact of forces upon form is also beautifully evidenced in the form of three different classes of creatures who came to live in the sea, as shown in Figure 4–9.

Abnormal mechanical forces give rise to deformation in man in much the same fashion as abnormal forces may deform a tree. In addition to those extrinsic deformations that relate to uterine constraint, this can be seen in the deformations wrought by past societies in the name of beauty or custom by application of external forces after the time of birth, as shown in Figure 4–10*A* and *B*. Constraint forces were utilized to mold the head by a number of groups, including the "Flathead Indians," whose name derived from the practice. In the past the Chinese custom of binding the feet of infant girls resulted in small and misshapen feet. In some societies the insertion of stretching devices into the ear lobes resulted in excessive skin in this region, as did similar practices with the lip. These techniques were designed to cause deformations. Other practices, such as the swaddling or papoose-board immobilization of infants, may have inadvertently increased the likelihood of deformation or hip dislocation.

Just as some past societies were knowledge-

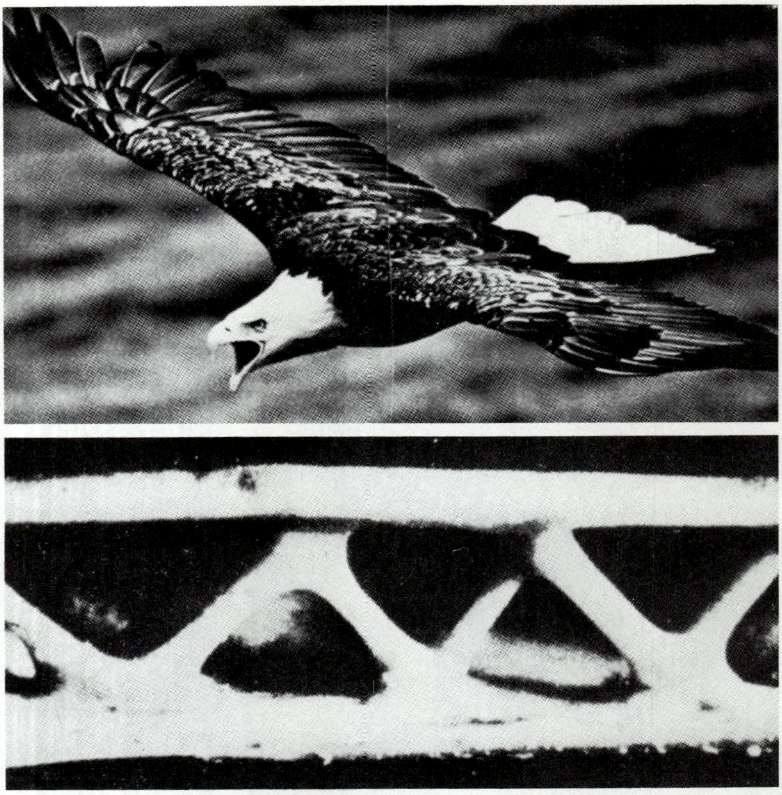

Figure 4–7. In the pneumatized bone in the wing of the soaring vulture, such as in the bald eagle (above), the orientation relates to the direction of air forces from below and above the wing. This generates a truss type of orientation highly similar to that utilized in the wing girders of early airplanes. (Bottom, from Thompson, d'Arcy: On Growth and Form. A New Edition. Cambridge. The University Press, 1942.)

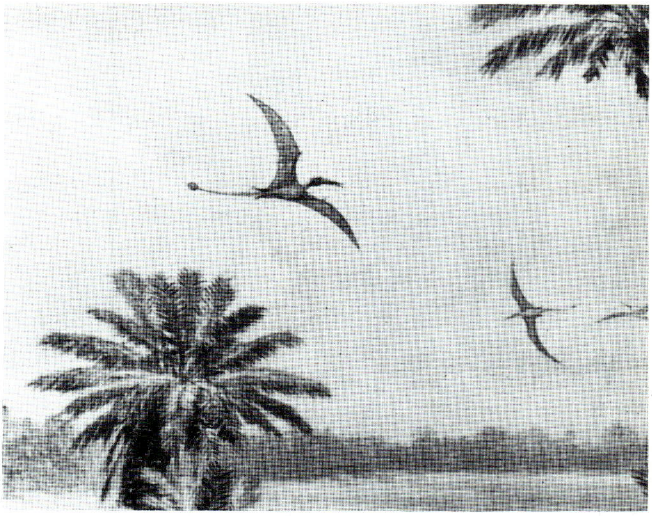

Figure 4–8. The form of the pteradon, related in ideal fashion to its function. (Courtesy of Ms. Pam Haas, American Museum of Natural History, New York City. Painting by Charles Wright.)

able about mechanical means of producing deformations after birth, so other societies successfully utilized biomechanical means to treat some congenital deformations. In India there are women who specialize in reshaping deformations by daily massage and manipulation. Among Polynesian societies, in which talipes equinovarus was a common deformity, there was usually an older woman who specialized in manipulating and binding such feet. The deformation was deliberately only partially corrected because such feet were ideal for climbing coconut trees and no shoes were needed in their environment!

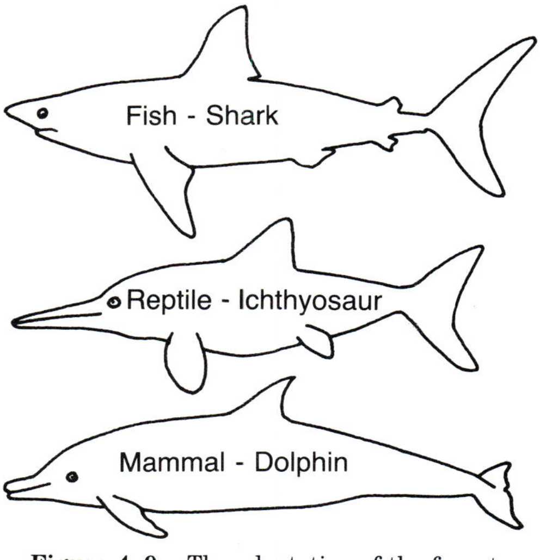

Figure 4–9. The adaptation of the form toward reducing turbulence and toward ease of free movement in water is beautifully exemplified by the similarities of form in a larger free swimming fish, a reptile, and a mammal. In this environment gravity is of less importance than is the buoyancy of the sea in shaping form.

(Adapted from Bunnell, S., and McIntyre, J.: Mind in the Waters. New York, Charles Scribner & Sons, 1974.)

MECHANICAL IMPACTS ON MORPHOGENESIS

Mechanical forces play an important role in the normal morphogenesis of most tissues. Particular tissues have their own limited repertoire of responses to forces. The abnormalities mentioned in this section are utilized predominantly to more dramatically illustrate mechanical hypotheses that are relevant to normal morphogenesis of particular tissues. Many of the examples relate to the impact of forces during early morphogenesis, when extrinsic constraint deformation would be unlikely to occur. However, they do provide the reader with some clinically relevant illustrations of the impact of forces on form in morphogenesis.

Overall Growth

Constraint may limit the growth of the whole individual.[2] When the onset of constraint growth deficiency occurs during late fetal life there will usually be catch-up growth into the normal range once the constraint is relieved following birth. This appears to be the reason why the first born, who must distend out the uterus and the mother's abdominal wall for the first time, averages about 200 to 300 gm smaller than subsequent offspring. The more the constraint, the greater is the deceleration of growth. This is dramatically evident in most multiple births. As shown in Figure 3–11, page 105, twins grow at a normal rate for the first 30 to 34 weeks of gestation. After they have achieved a combined weight of 4.0 kg, they become constrained and the growth rate tends to slow. The same types of phenomena have been

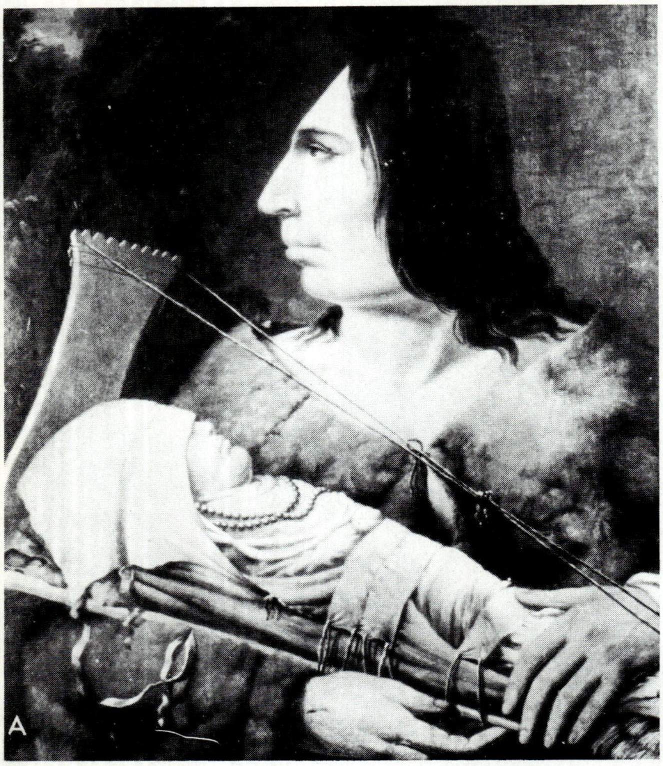

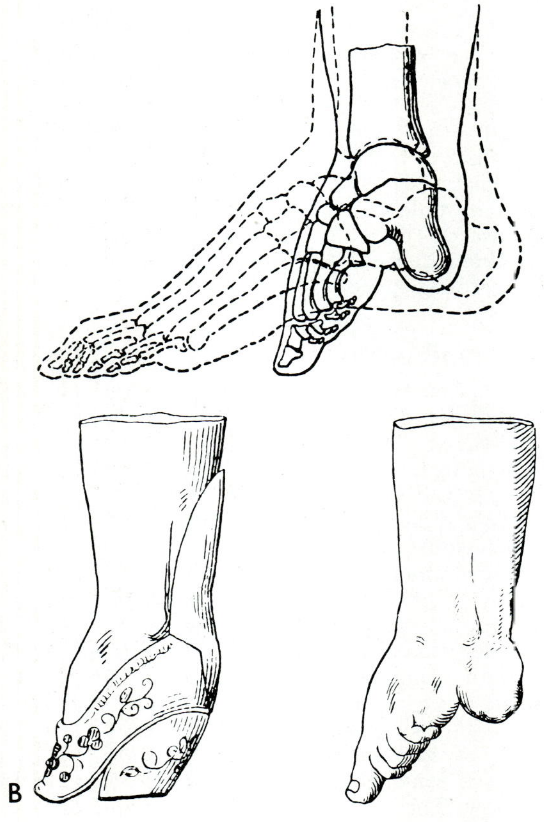

Figure 4–10. *A,* The Kwakiutl American Indians of the Northwest utilized cedar boards and leather tongs to mold the infant heads. Boys were molded for five months and girls were generally molded for seven months. (Courtesy of Bill Holm, the Burke Memorial Washington State Museum.)

B, For almost 1500 years certain young Chinese girls were subjected to harrowing molding for a matter of years in order to produce small feet. These feet were deemed sexually attractive. The form into which the deformed feet were molded is shown above and the special shoe and foot position is shown below. (From Levy, H.S.: Chinese Footbinding. New York, Walton Rawls, 1966.)

noted in animal studies. If only one animal is reared in a uterine horn, the newborn is appreciably larger at birth than when many are reared in the same uterine horn.[3]

There are many other situations besides multiple births that limit the intrauterine space, causing it to yield a smaller baby. Examples include oligohydramnios, uterine malformation, and uterine fibroids. An example of the latter is shown in Figure 4–11.

Effects on Specific Tissues

Bone. The early cartilage models of the long bones appear to be genetically determined, but the alignment of collagen fibrils and of bone trabeculae relate to mechanical forces, as do the bony promontories. The alignment of collagen fibrils in the same direction as stress forces, thereby avoiding shear forces, has already been alluded to, as has the impact of the sites of muscle attachment on bone form. For example, the size and shape of the greater trochanter relates to the rather massive pull of five muscles at that site, including the very strong gluteus maximus muscle. The lesser trochanter has only one major muscle attaching at that site, the psoas minor. The combined forces of weight bearing plus muscle pull affect the form of the upper femur,

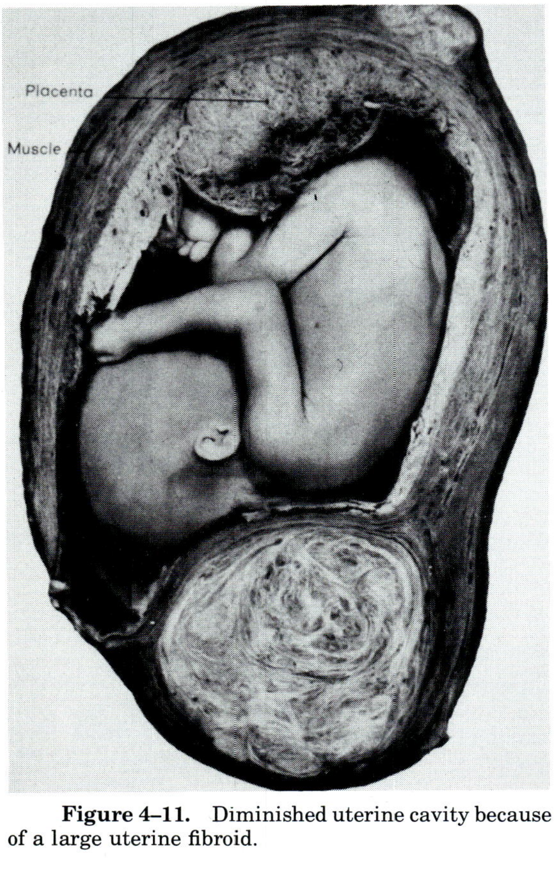

Figure 4–11. Diminished uterine cavity because of a large uterine fibroid.

including the normal "neck" of the femur. Prolonged muscle weakness in the growing child may give rise to less prominence of the trochanters and a straighter neck of the femur, a so-called coxa valga, as shown in Figure 4–12. It is important that these bony findings be interpreted as secondary deformations, the consequence of a more primary neuromuscular problem, rather than as additional malformations involving the skeletal system.

The impact of increasing weight is also evident on the breadth of bone. The strength of a leg bone, for example, depends on the area of its cross section. Since the legs must hold up a body that increases in weight by the cube of its height, they thicken much more in a heavy person than they do in a small person. Galileo first recognized this principle in his *Discorsi* in 1638. He reasoned that the bone of a large animal must thicken disproportionately in order to provide the same relative strength as the slender bone of a small animal.

Stress forces affect not only the form of bone but also the growth of bone. Linear growth is only mildly affected by muscle weakness. Thus, paralysis of a limb results in only a 5 to 10 per cent reduction in its rate of linear growth. However, subperiosteal growth in bone breadth is more dramatically affected. Hence, with muscle weakness or lack of use, the growing bone tends to become slender, as is shown in Figure 4–13.

The adaptive capacity of bone is beautifully exemplified by the realization that the amount of bone present and its alignment are influenced by the very forces that the bone is required to withstand. Bone appears to have a critical strain or stress threshold above which there tends to be bone deposition and below which there tends to be bone resorption. Intermittent stress on a bone tends to foster local growth of bone, as exemplified in bony promontories at sites of muscle attachment. One example is the bony spurs that are liable to develop in the arch of the foot as a result of the strain of long distance running. However, persistent stress on a bone, such as is caused by continuous external compression, can lead to a decrease in bone. This is dramatically exemplified by constraint vertex craniotabes. This abnormality appears most commonly to be secondary to prolonged constraint pressure on the fetal head as a consequence of the head being forcibly "engaged" for a long period of time prior to birth.

A similar but postnatal type of impact of persisting pressure on the calvarium was deduced by G. E. Smith[4] from his evaluation of ancient Egyptian skulls. He recognized that the upper class Egyptians who lived during the fourth to the nineteenth dynasties and who wore heavy wigs had a peculiar thinning of the calvarium. Smith deduced that this was the consequence of the *continuous pressure* exerted by these heavy head pieces!

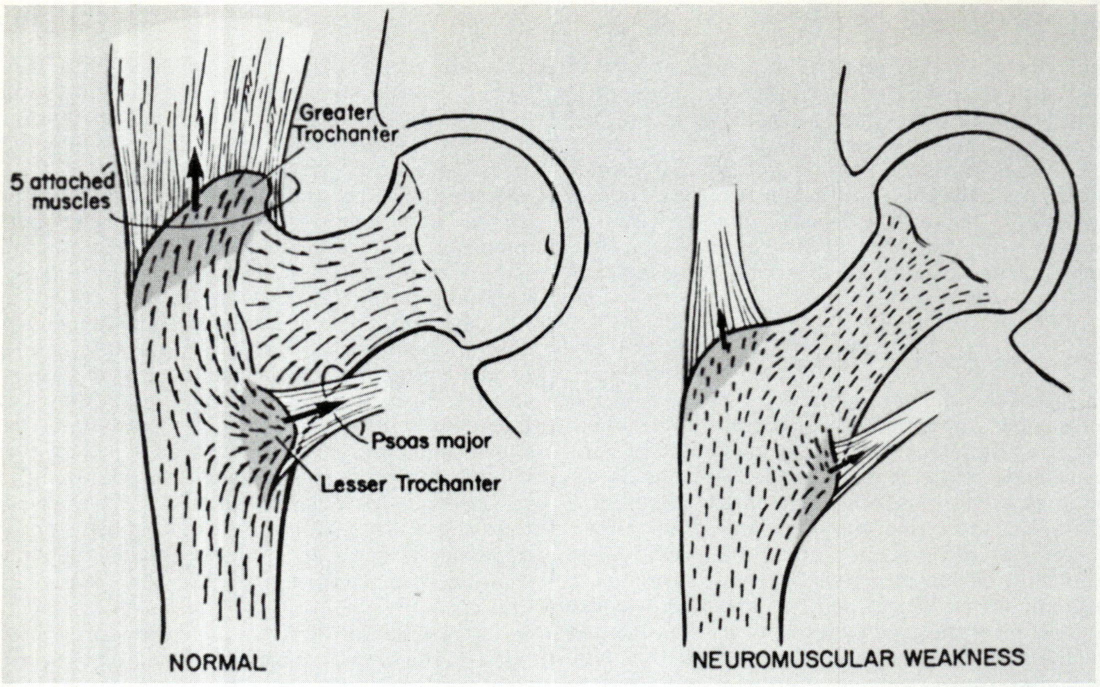

Figure 4–12. Impact of muscle weakness on the form of the proximal femur. The coxa valga and slimmer bone is secondary to the diminished forces exerted on the bone.

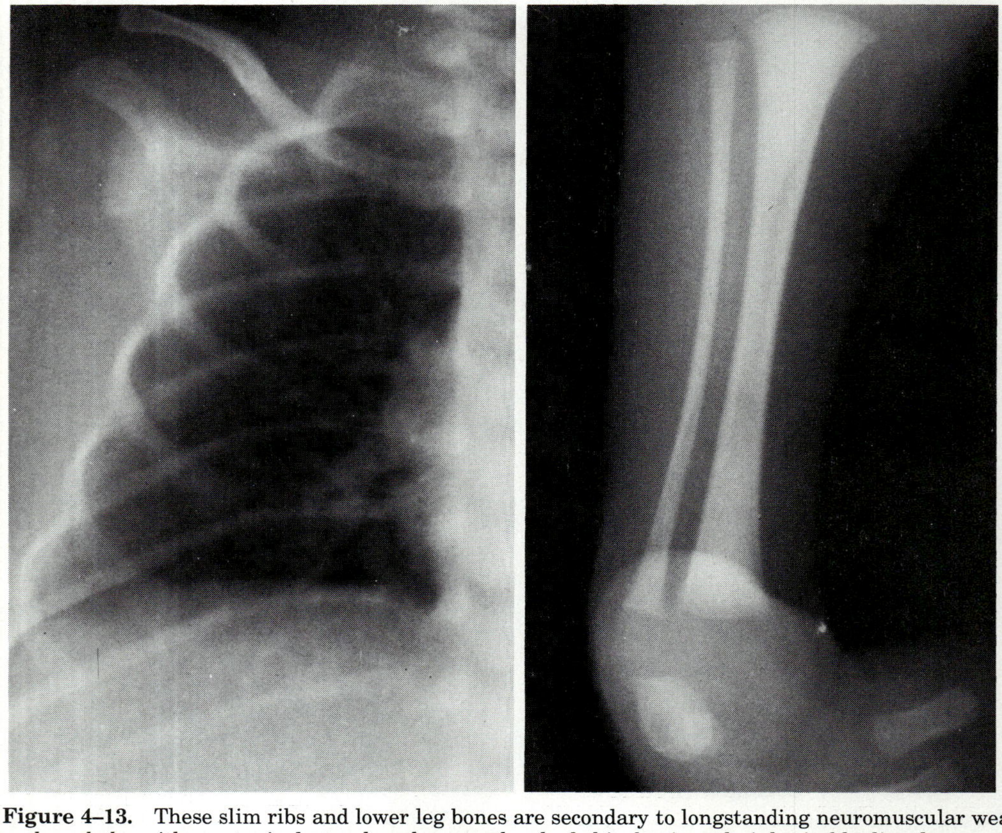

Figure 4–13. These slim ribs and lower leg bones are secondary to longstanding neuromuscular weakness in a newborn baby with myotonic dystrophy whose mother had this dominantly inheritable disorder.

Joints. Joints develop secondarily within the condensed mesenchyme of the developing bones. Movement is an important factor in joint morphogenesis. A chronic lack of movement tends to give rise to joint contracture.[5] One dramatic example was an infant with multiple joint contractures (termed arthrogryposis) whose mother had received tubocurarine for 19 days in early pregnancy for the treatment of tetanus.[6] The medically induced early immobilization for 19 days was considered to be the cause of the joint contractures in the fetus. Physical constraint may also yield joint contracture.

Muscles. Muscle cells align in the direction of muscle pull. In addition to avoiding shear forces, this has obvious importance to muscle function. The size of the muscle relates to the magnitude and frequency of the forces: the larger the forces, the greater is the muscle bulk. Conversely, with diminished function, the muscles become smaller in size. A lack of any function will result in a diminished, hypoplastic muscle. The biomechanical impact of muscle strength on bone form and growth has already been emphasized.

Organ Capsules. Organ capsules may be viewed as exoskeletons that provide connective tissue support for particular tissues. Included within this category are the dura mater of the brain, the sclera and outer covering of the eye, the pericardium of the heart, the pleura of the lung, the peritoneum of the intestine, the capsule of the kidney, and the tunica albuginea of the testes. The skin may also be interpreted as an organ capsule: it is the capsule for the entire organism. The only organ capsule that becomes ossified is that of the brain. The dura mater is responsible for the development and ossification of the calvarium; this will be considered in more depth in the craniofacial section. None of these organ capsules appear to have any basic impetus for growth. Rather, they grow in accordance with the mechanical forces imposed by the expansion of the particular organ or tissue that they envelop. All the organ capsules are composed of connective tissues within which the collagen fibrils align in accordance with the growth stretch imposed by the internal expansile growth of the respective organ. The direction of such forces is curvilinear, as is readily evident in the alignment of the collagen fibrils within these organ capsules.

Skin and Its Derivatives. Skin does not appear to have any basic impetus for growth, but grows in accordance with mechanical forces.[7] Normally the forces are exerted by the growth of underlying tissues. If there is unusual growth of underlying tissues, the skin will respond accordingly. Thus, if there is hydrocephalus, the skin will grow in accordance with the enlarged head. The excessive skin of the "web neck" which may occur in XO Turner syndrome and other disorders is considered secondary to a more primary problem in the development of the lymphatic system, as shown in Figure 4–14. A defect in communication between the jugular lymph sac and the internal jugular vein results in a grossly distended jugular lymph sac which increases the growth of the skin in that posterolateral region of the neck. The lymphaticovenous communication usually develops before the time of birth, thus draining the distended lymphatic sacs. The excess skin remains as a redundant fold from the mastoid region toward the shoulder, a deformational clue to the nature of the problem that engendered the "web neck." Another condition that may leave a residuum of redundant skin is early urethral obstruction, which can massively distend the bladder in early fetal life. This will usually be lethal early in fetal life unless the bladder decompresses, which will yield a wrinkled "prune belly" with redundant folds of abdominal skin at birth.

The skin appears to respond to external pressure by growth in a fashion similar to its response to internal expansile stretch. For example, when there has been external constraint on the skin, such as with oligohydramnios, there may be loose and redundant folds of skin at birth. Such accentuated folds in the face may account for the "Potter facies" noted with the external constraint due to oligohydramnios. I have noted redundant loose folds on the back of the neck in infants who have been in prolonged breech presentation with the head hyperextended to yield the "breech head" deformation. This is presumed to be the consequence of excessive pressure of the basiocciput on the posterior neck resulting in localized overgrowth of the skin in this region. In similar fashion, skin overgrowth in an anterior neck and chin region may be noted with prolonged face presentation. Thus, the finding of redundant excessive skin at birth may implicate either past internal expansile growth stretch or past external compressive constraint of considerable duration.

An occasional finding in a normal baby is a small raw, punched-out lesion in the skin of the scalp. Such lesions also are a frequent feature in babies with the 13 trisomy syndrome, as shown in Figure 4–15, and occasionally in other disorders. They tend to occur in close proximity to the parietal hair whorl. It is the contention of the author that the parietal hair whorl represents the apical point from which growth stretch is exerted by the domelike outgrowth of the brain. This point in the developing skin of the scalp would therefore be the most liable to break down during the period of rapid brain growth which stretches the skin away from this point. Under this hypothesis, the ulceration would be the result of the interaction of mechanical forces plus a greater than average liability to breakdown of the skin at this point of maximal stretch.

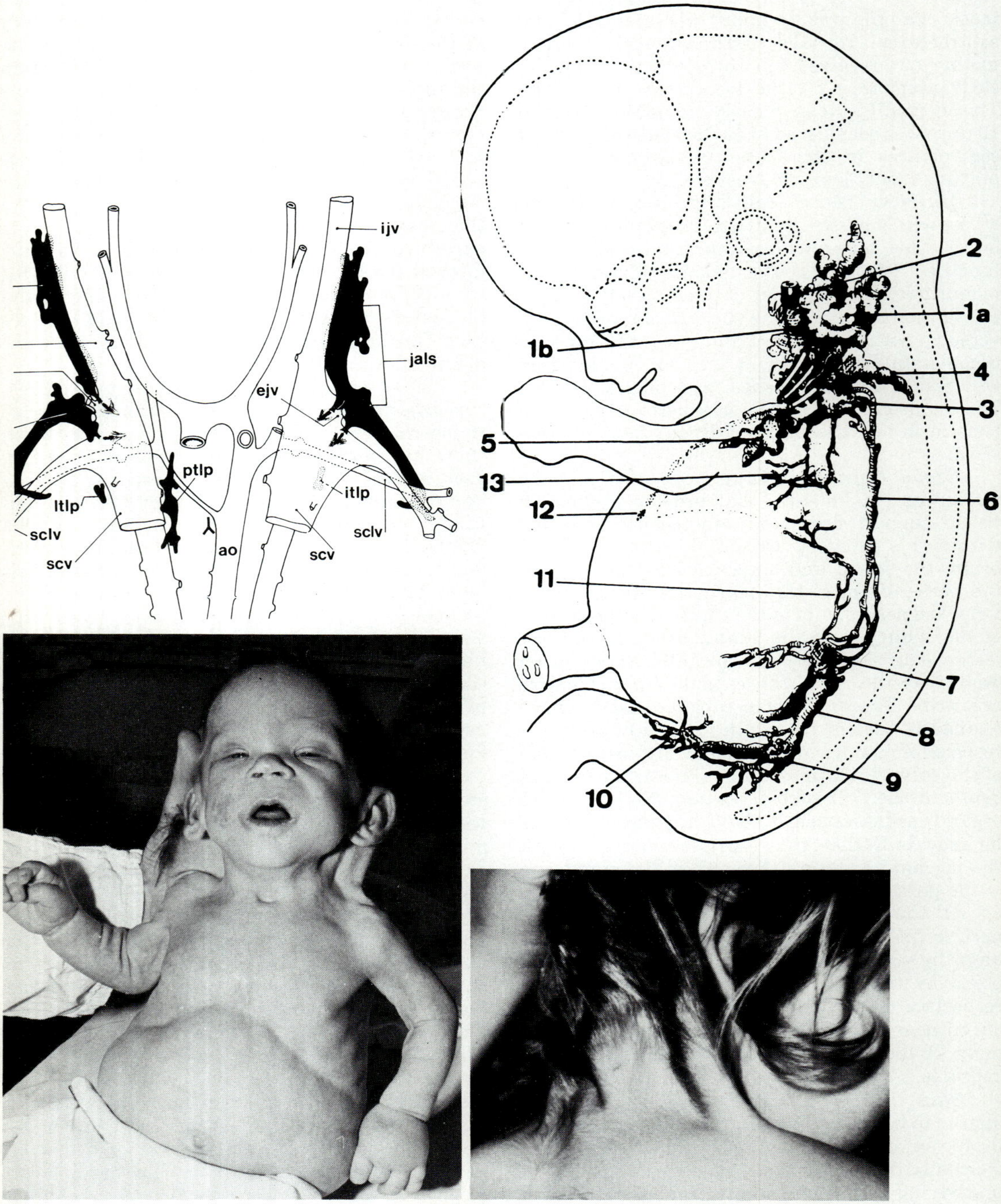

Figure 4–14. See legend on opposite page

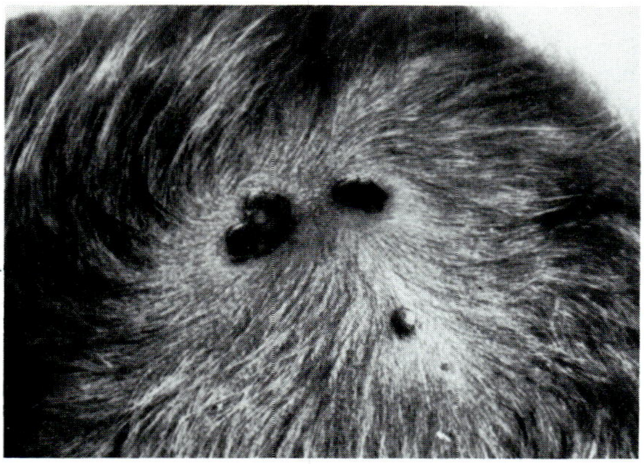

Figure 4-15. Small scalp ulcerations in a newborn infant with the 13 trisomy syndrome. Note that these lesions tend to occur at or near the site of the parietal hair whorl, the location of maximal stretch exerted on the developing skin of the scalp by the domelike outgrowth of the brain.

1. Hair directional patterning: As the hair follicles are down-growing from the germinative layer of the skin at 10 to 18 weeks of development they come to have a sloping angulation (Fig. 4-16).[8] This angulation is considered to be the consequence of the direction and magnitude of growth stretch exerted on the surface skin during the period of downgrowth of the hair follicles which as a result of differential lag have a sloping angulation. When the keratinized rod of hair is finally extruded at 18 weeks of development, its hair direction appears to be set for life and reflects the magnitude and direction of growth stretch exerted on the skin during the 11 to 18 week fetal period (Figs. 4-17 and 4-18). On any expanding sphere or hemisphere there is one immobile point away from which all other points are moving. Over the scalp this is usually in the parietal region and is considered the genesis of the parietal hair whorl, or crown. This is a beautiful example of the impact of mechanical forces on form. Thus differences in brain growth and form are considered the reason for most differences in scalp hair directional patterning, including those that exist between humans and other primates, as shown in Figure 4-19. Of special clinical relevance are the aberrant hair directional patterns that may be secondary to problems of brain morphogenesis, examples of which are shown in Figures 4-20 through 4-23. Such findings not only tend to implicate a problem in brain morphogenesis but also suggest that the disorder had its advent prior to 16 weeks of fetal life.

2. Nails: Each nail is a keratinized plate which, as with hair follicles, is derived from the germinative layer of skin. The nail tends to conform to the shape of the distal phalanx, as shown in Figure 4-24. Thus, if the distal phalanx is short and broad, the nail is short and broad. If the distal phalanx is narrow, the nail is narrow. The impact of forces on the early form of the nails is illustrated in Figure 4-25.

3. Dermal ridge patterning: As with other primates, man has dermal ridges on the thickened skin of the volar surface of the hand and foot. This parallel ridging provides an important frictional surface for the palm and sole. These ridges develop at 13 to 19 weeks of fetal life and appear to form at right angles to the plane of growth stretch in the skin.[9] Figure 4-26 illustrates the similarity to the ridges that develop in the sand of a beach at right angles to the direction of the flow of water or of wind. The surface characteristics where there are underlying pads give rise to curvilinear dermal ridge patterns that reflect the shape of the pads at the time of dermal ridge development (Figs. 4-27 and 4-28). If the fingertip pad were low, the patterning would be an arch. However, if the pads were very prominent, a whorl would be expected, with the

---

Figure 4-14. *Upper right,* The early developing lymph channels drain into the venous system. In the cervical region the jugular lymph sac (1a) drains into the jugular vein (2) at the site designated 1b. This is shown in the upper left at 40 days of development, by which time the communication (arrows) from the jugular and axillary lymph sacs (jals) has occurred into the jugular vein.

Upper left, If there is a delay or failure in the development of the communication between the lymphatic system and the venous system there is a damming up of the lymph, as was still evident at the time of birth in this XO Turner syndrome girl. The distended jugular lymph sac results in the growth of excess skin in the lateral neck. Once the lymph drainage has occurred, the individual is left with a residuum of redundant skin referred to as "web neck," shown at lower right in the same girl several years later. Lymph accumulation may yield peripheral lymphedema, and prior lymph accumulation may yield such residual features as loose skin in the face and a lax abdomen. (Upper right from Töndury, G., and Kubik, S.: Zur ontogenese des lymphatischen Systems. Handbuch der Allgemeinen Pathologie, Berlin, Springer-Verlag, 1975. Upper left from van der Putte, S.C.: The development of the lymphatic system in man. Adv. Anat. Embryol. *51*:1, 1975.)

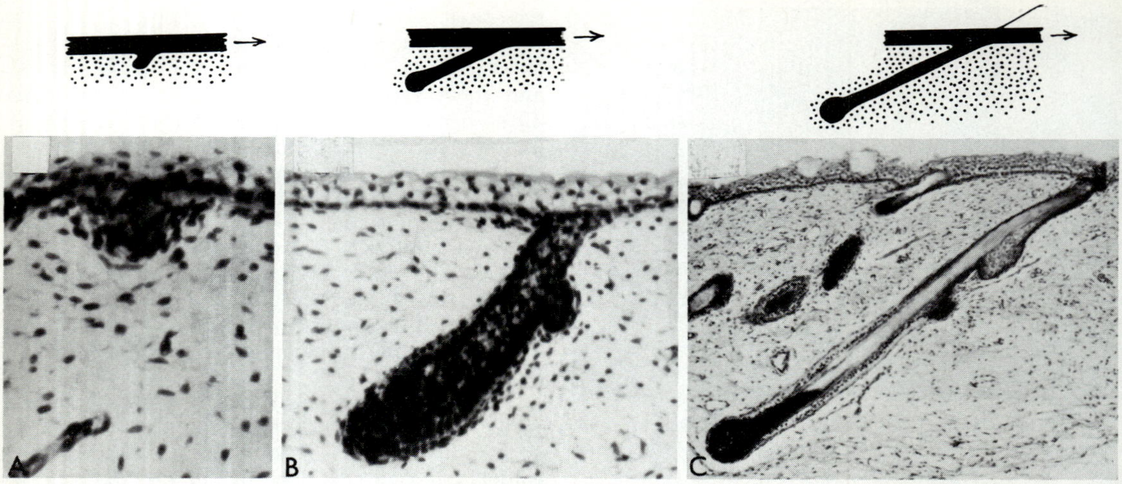

Figure 4–16. As a hair follicle grows downward, its direction of angulation is determined by the forces exerted via the underlying growth of the brain. These stretch forces, greater at the surface than in deeper tissues, affect the hair directional patterning, which is usually set by about 16 weeks. (From Smith, D.W., and Gong, B.T.: Teratology *9*:17, 1974.)

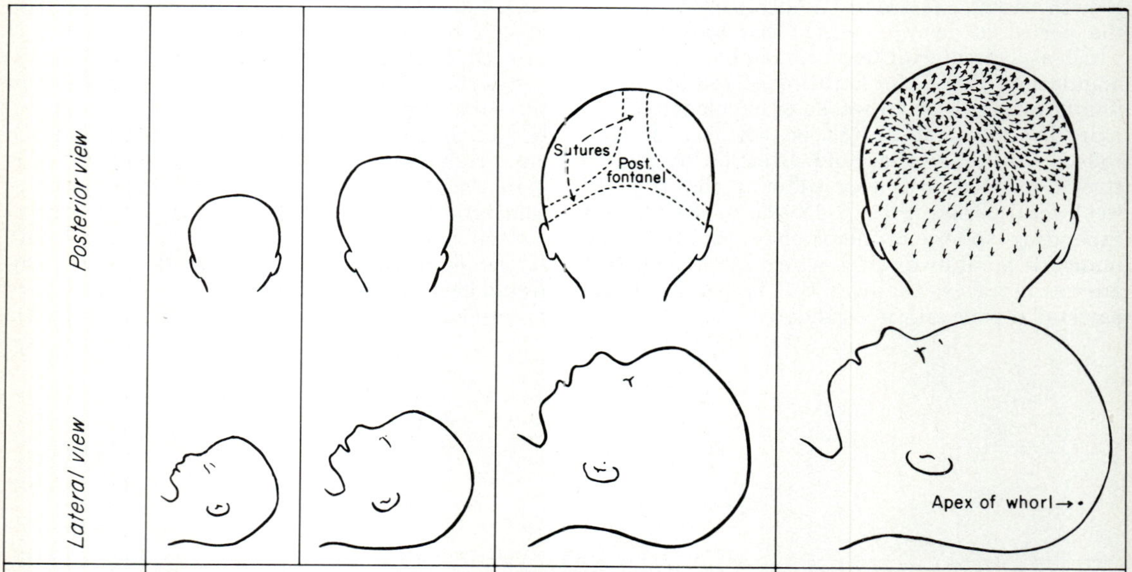

Hair	Early hair follicles with sloping downgrowth		Hair being produced	Surface hair patterning evident
Gestational age	11 weeks	12 ½ weeks	16 ½ weeks	18 weeks
C-R length	71 mm	83 mm	122 mm	145 mm

Figure 4–17. The rapid domelike projection of the brain during the period of hair follicle downgrowth is evident in these proportionate drawings of the early fetal head, during the era of hair follicle downgrowth. (From Smith, D.W., and Gong, B.T.: Teratology *9*:17, 1974.)

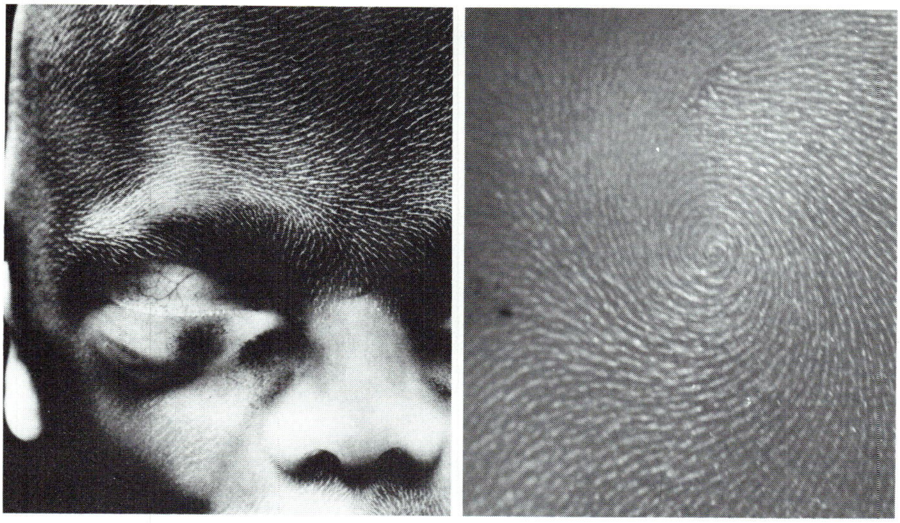

Figure 4–18. As the hairs emerge at about 18 weeks the hair directional patterns are beautifully evident. *Left,* Over the forehead the "frontal hair stream," emanating from the fixed skin points of the ocular puncta, meets with the downsweeping parietal hair stream, which emanates from the parietal whorl. *Right,* The parietal hair whorl (crown). On any expanding sphere or hemisphere there must be at least one fixed point from which all other points are moving. Presumably it is the mild asymmetry of forces which conveys the whorl pattern. (From Smith, D.W., and Gong, B.T.: Teratology *9*:17, 1974.)

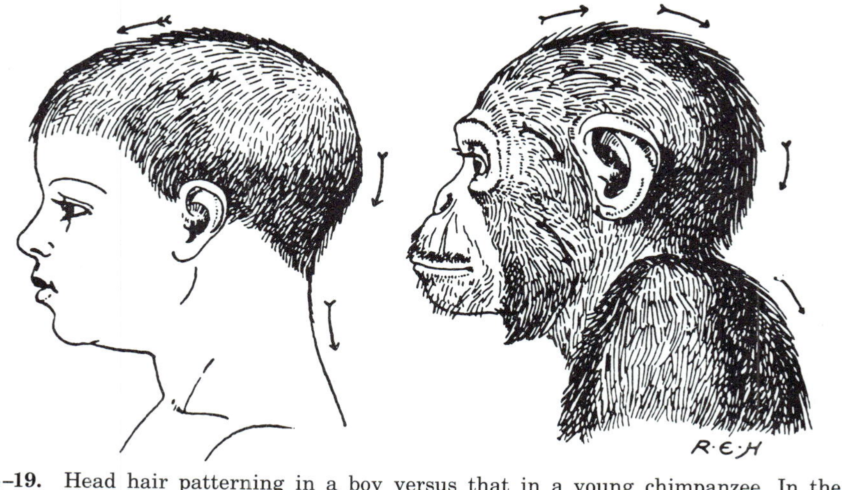

Figure 4–19. Head hair patterning in a boy versus that in a young chimpanzee. In the human, the large domelike brain has generated a parietal whorl and the hair "streams" from that spot, with the parietal hair stream sweeping forward to meet with the frontal hair stream on the forehead. Since the chimpanzee has a much smaller brain, the frontal hair stream simply sweeps directly back over the head with no parietal whorl or parietal hair stream. (From Kidd, W.: The Direction of Hair in Animals and Man. London, Adam and Charles Black, 1903.)

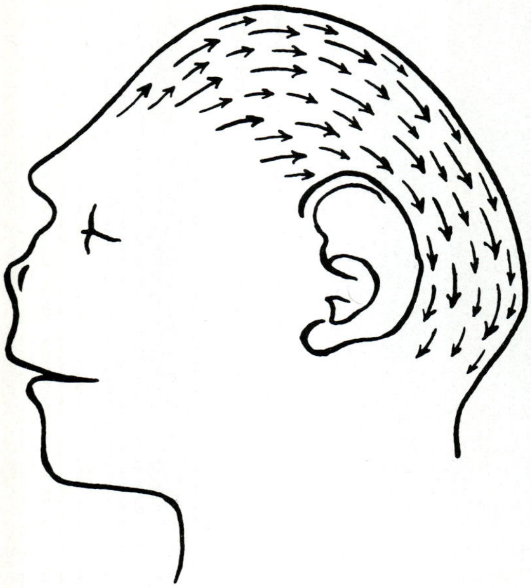

Figure 4–20. Child with severe microcephaly and mid-facial defect. There is no parietal hair whorl and the frontal hair stream sweeps back over the scalp in similar fashion to that found in the chimpanzee (Figure 4–19). (From Smith, D.W., and Gong, B.T.: Teratology *9*:17, 1974.)

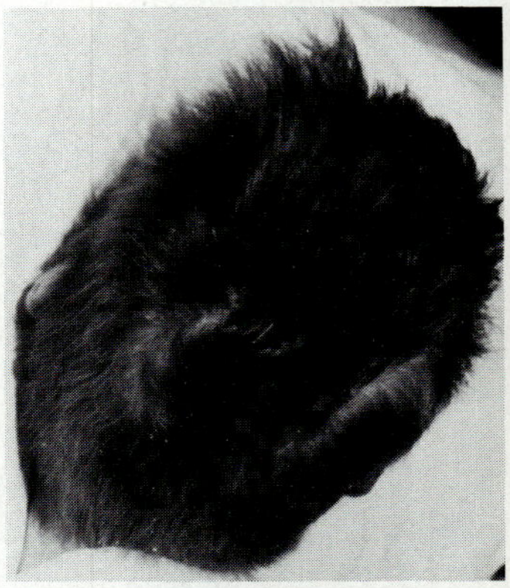

Figure 4–21. Lack of a definitive posterior whorl in a child with severe microcephaly. (From Smith, D.W., and Gong, B.T.: Teratology *9*:17, 1974.)

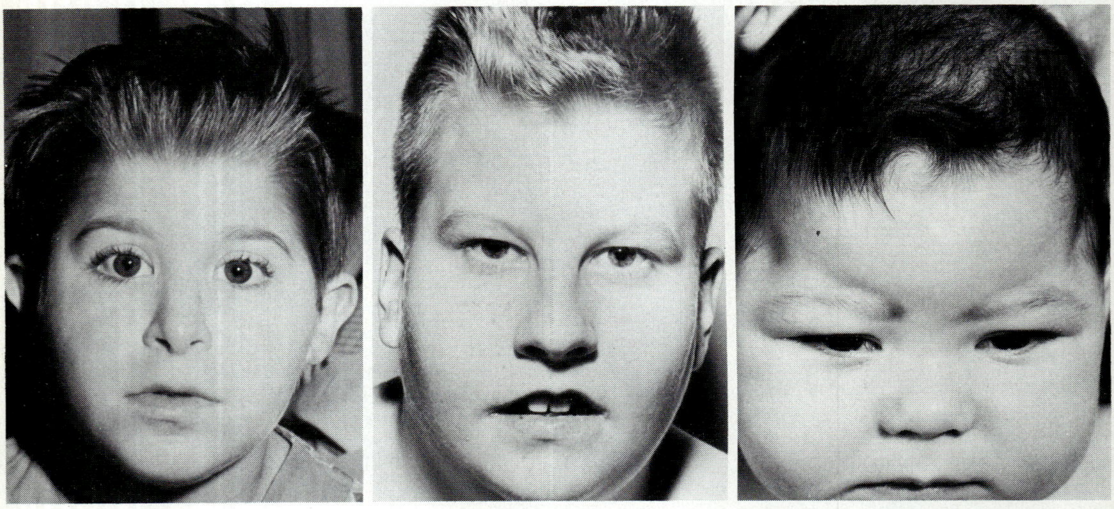

Figure 4–22. Frontal brain deficiency may result in the frontal hair stream sweeping upward into the scalp region and giving rise to a frontal upsweep, more commonly refered to as a "cowlick." Mild degrees of this occur in about 3 per cent of normal individuals. These represent unusual degrees in a child with Rubinstein-Taybi syndrome (left), Prader-Willi syndrome (middle), and fetal rubella syndrome (right). At the site of juncture of the upsweeping frontal hair stream and the downsweeping parietal hair stream there may be a convergent whorl, as shown to the right. (Left and middle from Smith, D.W., and Gong, B.T.: Teratology *9*:17, 1974. Right, courtesy of Dr. Patrick MacLeod, University of British Columbia.)

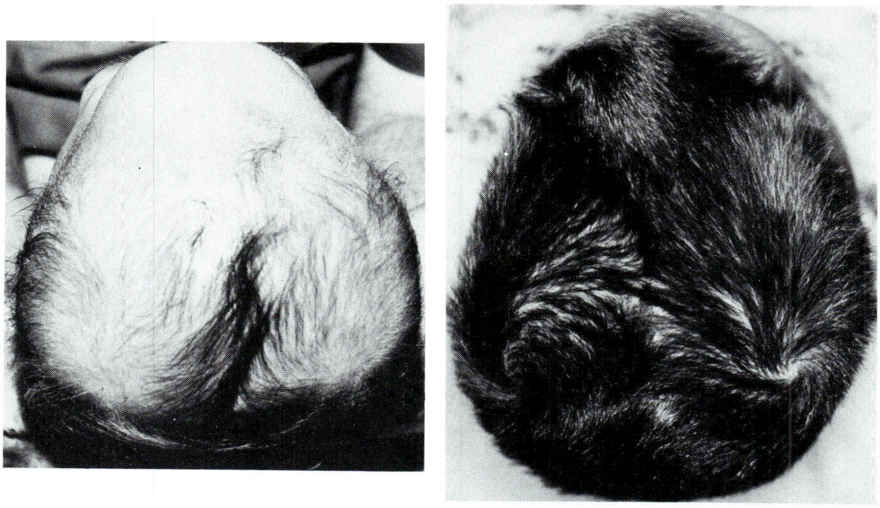

Figure 4–23. Two children with trigonocephaly. The wide placement of two parietal whorls is compatible with the developing brain having had an abnormal triangular shape prior to 16 weeks of fetal life. Five per cent of normal children have bilateral parietal whorls, but they are spaced close to the midline in contrast to the situation in these two individuals. (From Smith, D.W., and Gong, B.T.: Teratology *9*:17, 1974.)

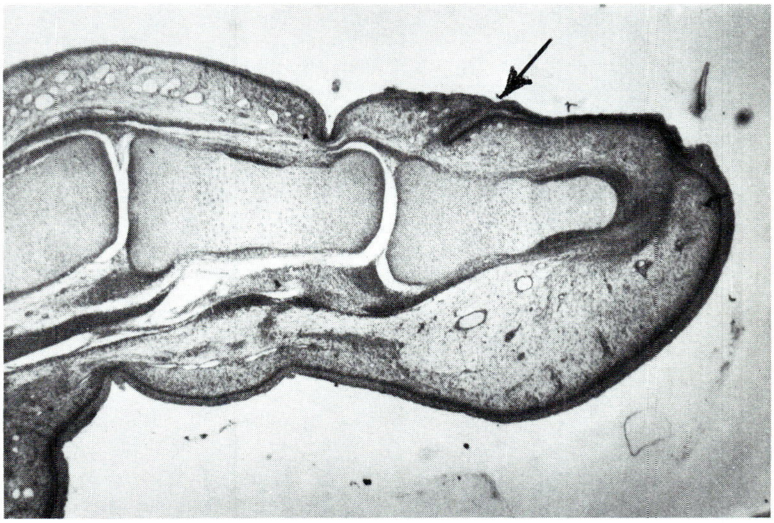

Figure 4–24. Longitudinal section of the finger in an 11 week fetus showing the orientation of the early nail plate (arrow) to the distal phalanx. The growing cells of the nail plate become a keratinized nail which generally reflects the form of the underlying distal bony phalanx. (From Prof. Gian Töndury, University of Zurich.)

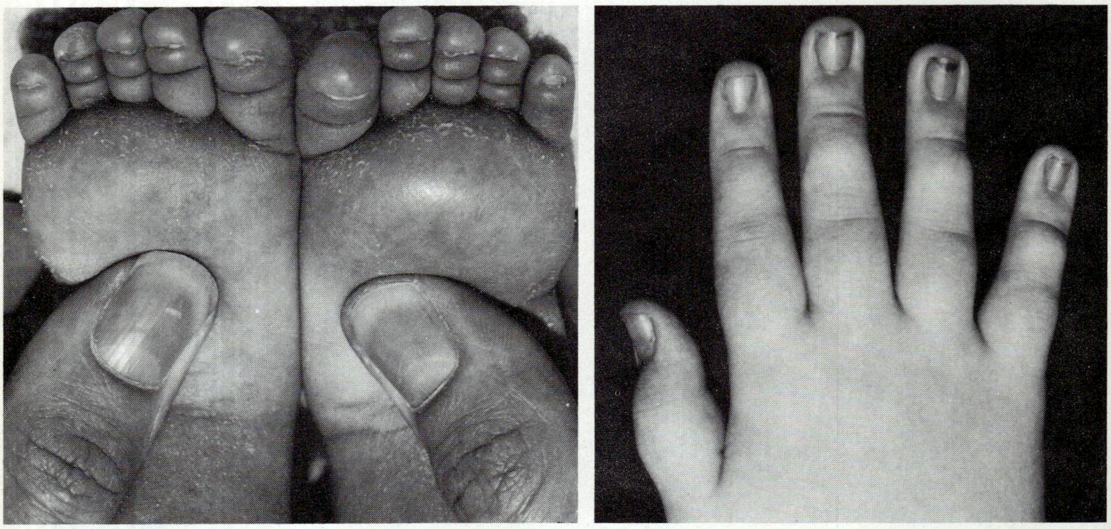

Figure 4–25. Fetal lymphedema may distort the form of the nails, as exemplified in a newborn and a child with peripheral lymphedema as one feature of the XO Turner syndrome. The narrow, hyperconvex nails with the appearance of a deep-set nail base are the residual consequences of prior lymphedema.

Figure 4–26. The ridges in the sand were generated at right angles to the direction of flow of water (above) and wind (below). Where there are undulations in the surface, the forces generate curvilinear patterns. Dermal ridges seem to be determined in somewhat similar fashion, tending to be at right angles to the direction of growth stretch.

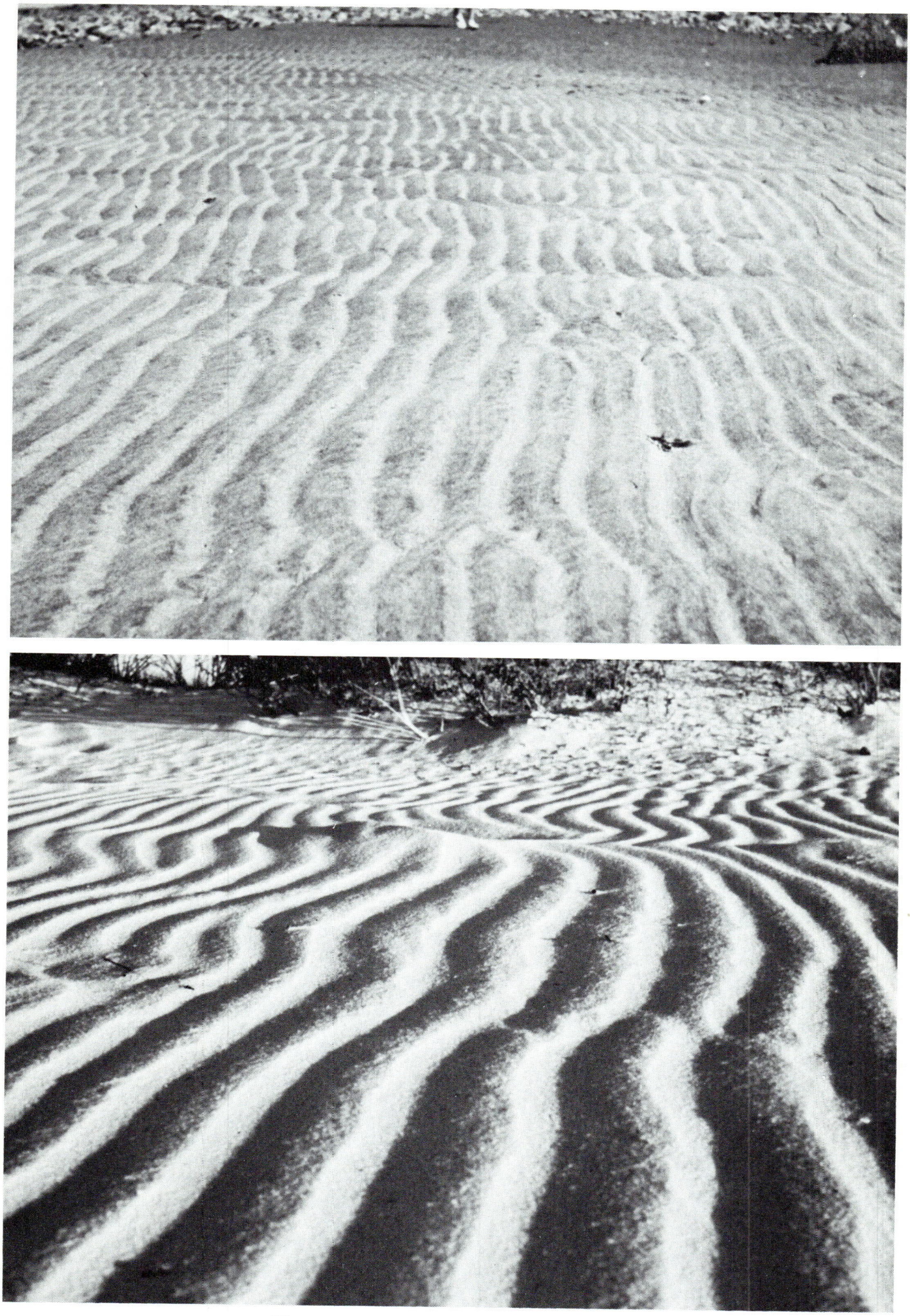

Figure 4–26. See legend on opposite page

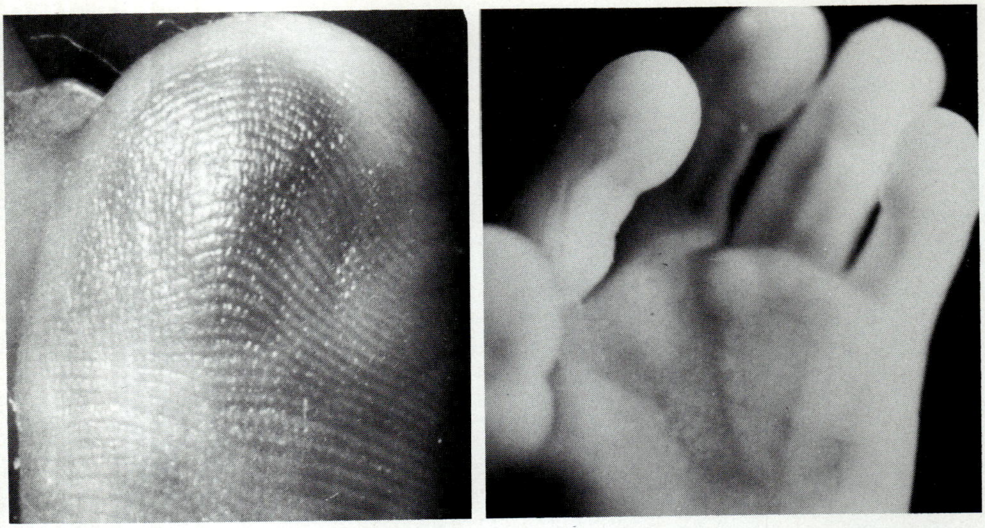

Figure 4–27. The dermal ridges, shown here on the distal finger of an infant (left) tend to develop at right angles to the growth stretch exerted on the skin by the development of the underlying tissues. Where there are pads, such as those shown in the fingertips and interdigital areas of the palm of a 10 week fetus (right), these result in the development of curvilinear ridge patterns, such as the low arch pattern on the fingertip shown to the left.

center of the whorl representing the apex of the pad. A high proportion of loops, the more common fingertip patterning, is of little clinical relevance. The finding of six or more arches on the 10 fingertips is unusual (3 per cent of normal), and the finding of eight or more whorls on the fingertips is also unusual. Altered dermal ridge patterning is generally a nonspecific deformation, providing evidence of the nature of the topographical growth in the volar surfaces of the hands and feet at 13 to 19 fetal weeks.

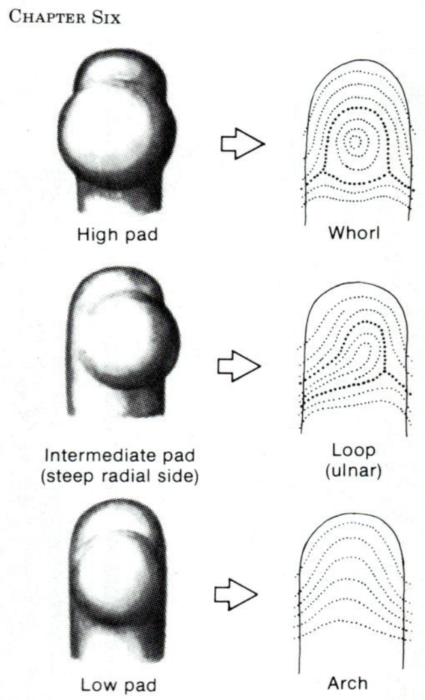

Figure 4–28. The fingertip dermal ridge patterning appears to relate to the form of the fingertip pads at the time of development of the dermal ridges. (From Mulvihill, J.J., and Smith, D.W.: J. Pediatr. *75*:579, 1969.)

4. Dermal creases: The dermal creases are simply deep wrinkles that reflect the flexional planes of functional folding in the thickened skin of the palms and soles,[10] as shown in Figure 4–29. They occur in relation to joints and provide evidence of the functional movement at such joints. Over the palm, the thenar flexional crease relates to the flexional plane of oppositional flexion of the thumb and first metacarpal. The upper palmar crease reflects the sloping plane of flexional folding of the third, fourth, and fifth metacarpophalangeal joints, and the mid-palmar crease simply reflects the folding plane in the skin between the other two palmar creases. By ever so small a difference in the shape or form of the hand it is possible to have a single upper palmar crease — the simian crease, as shown in Figure 4–30. This highly nonspecific finding is unilateral in 4 per cent of normals and bilateral in 1 per cent.

Craniofacial Region. The usual formation of the brain would appear to be of fundamental genetic determination. The growth of the brain in size (magnitude) and shape (direction) exerts a major mechanical impact on the form of the tissues that surround and relate to the brain in the craniofacial region. The early neural structures have the predominant impact. Thus, the brain affects the development of the calvarium and its sutures,[6] the optic cup evagination from the brain sets the stage for the orbit,[11] the invaginating neural olfactory placodes are primarily responsible for the subsequent formation of the nose and its accessories, and the invaginating auditory placode forms the inner ear and is responsible for much of the orientation of the temporal wing of the sphenoid bone. Therefore, the statement that the "face reflects the brain" has

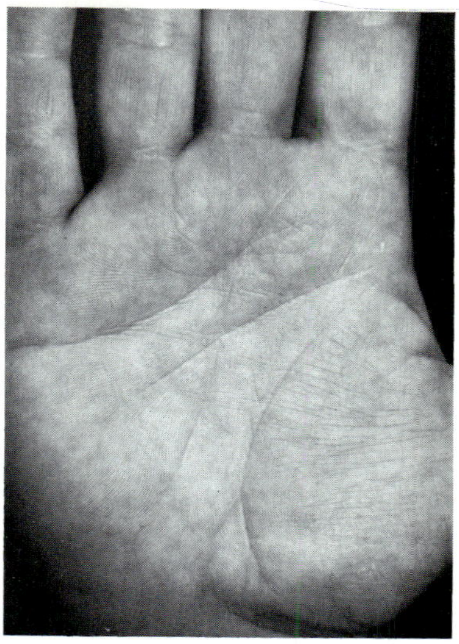

Figure 4–29. Creases relate to flexional planes of folding, always being secondary to mechanical forces. The upper palmar crease relates to the sloping plane of folding of the third, fourth, and fifth metacarpal-phalangeal joints, the thenar crease relates to the flexion of the thenar region, and the mid-palmar crease represents the folding plane between these two.

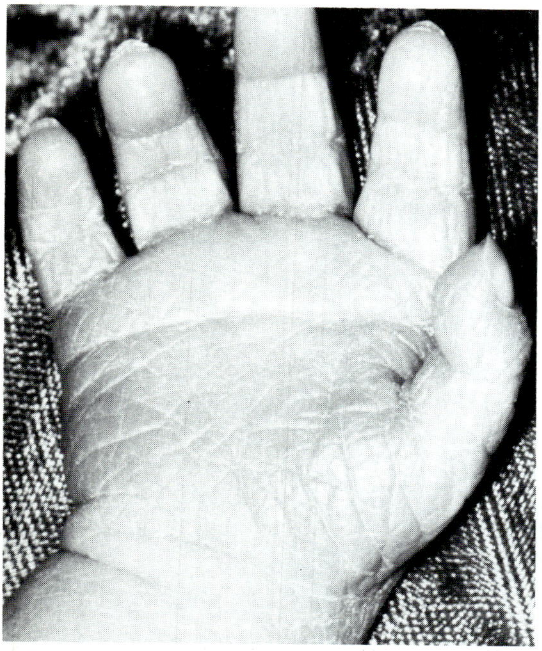

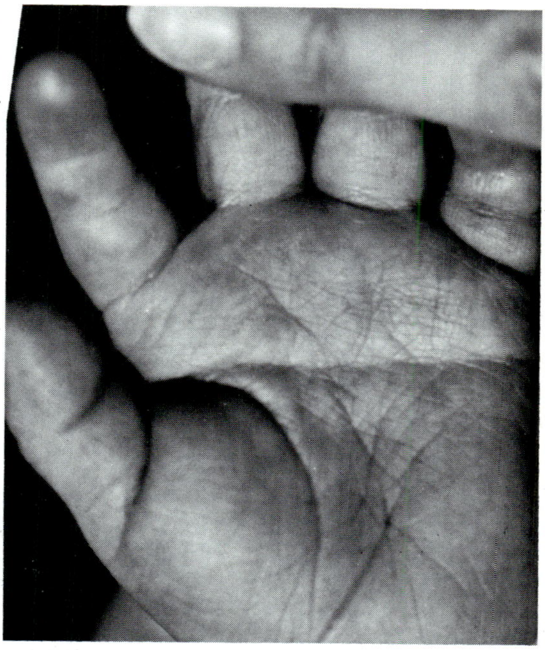

Figure 4–30. Minor differences in the form of the hand can result in a single crease across the upper palm (simian crease). The hand to the left has a short fifth finger and a single crease as a consequence. It also has an absence of the thenar crease, indicating a past functional deficit in oppositional flexional folding of the thenar region. The fine little creases occur when the skin of the hand is thin and have no further relevance.

much to support it. Particular features in the craniofacial region are summarized below.

Figures 4–31 and 4–32 emphasize the integral relationship that exists between the face and the brain. Beyond the mechanical impacts of brain development on facial form there are indirect effects of neuromuscular function on facial form. Such effects are depicted in Figures 4–33 and 4–34.

The Calvarium. It is the growth and shape of the brain that normally sets the form of the calvarium. Thus, in the absence of problems of calvarial development, such as constraint molding and/or craniostenosis, it is the brain that determines the shape of the calvarium. For example, a narrow forehead means a narrow forebrain, and a brachycephalic skull means a shorter length of brain.

The organ capsule of the brain, the dura mater, is literally the mother tissue in the development of the bony calvarium and its sutures (Figure 4–35). The calvarium *is* bone supported by strips of unmineralized dura, the sutures. These suture sites relate directly to the form of the early brain. As the brain grows outward, it balloons out the overlying dura mater. The brain is not a smooth hemisphere, and dural reflections occur into the recesses of the brain. The dural reflections are shown in Figure 4–36. Overlying these dural reflections, there is normally no ossification as long as there is continued growth stretch, as shown in Figure 4–37. These are the

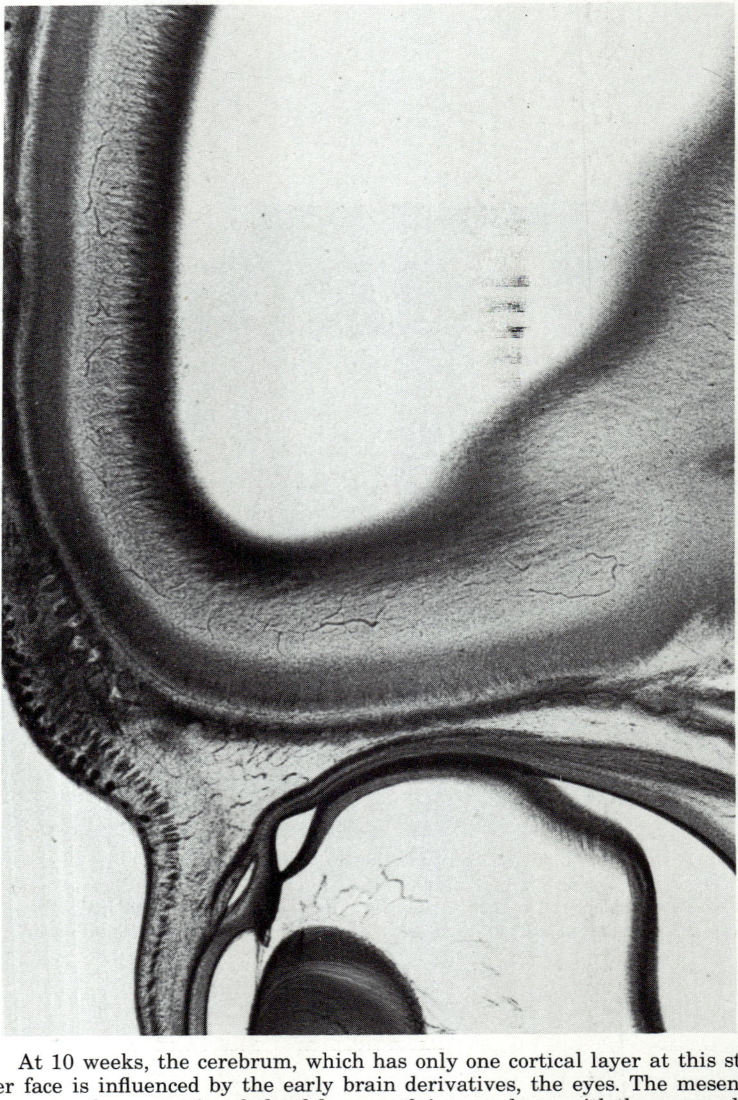

Figure 4–31. At 10 weeks, the cerebrum, which has only one cortical layer at this stage, is molding the forehead. The upper face is influenced by the early brain derivatives, the eyes. The mesenchymal tissues will soon condense and organize the supportive skeletal framework in accordance with these neural tissues. The growth of the cranial base anterior to the pituitary will occur in relationship to the frontal growth of the brain.

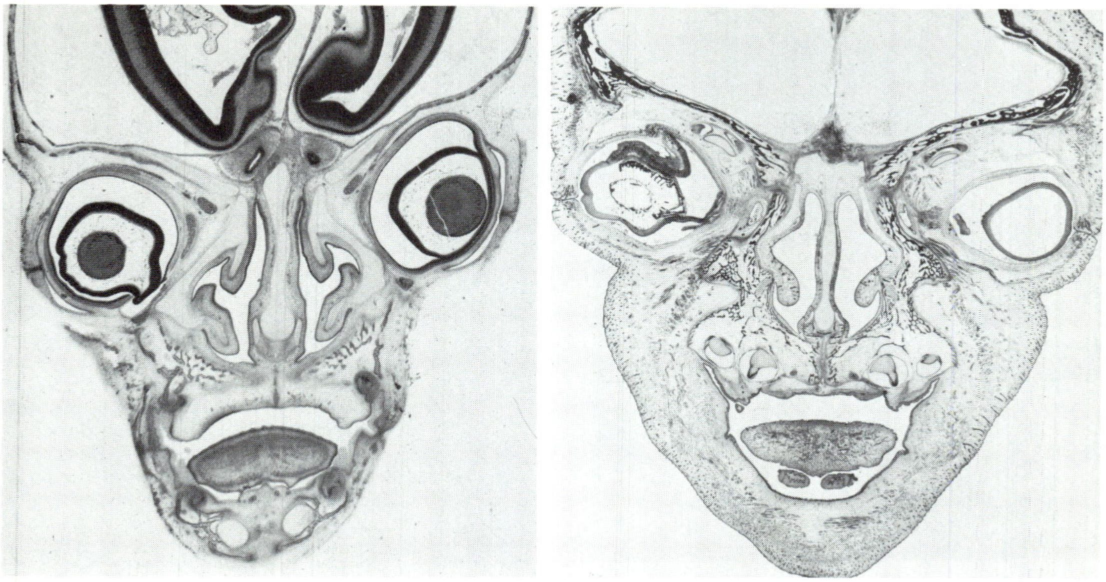

Figure 4–32. At 11 weeks (left) the relationship between the brain (contracted by fixation), the eyes, and the now cartilaginous upper facial skeleton is beautifully evident. This is also evident at 20 weeks (right, with brain removed), by which time much of the non-midline facial skeleton is ossified. Note the continuity between the cranial base and the facial skeleton. The anterior base of the brain *is* the roof of the face. (Left, from the Armed Forces Institute of Pathology, negative #76-5996. Right, from Burdi, A.R.: Early development of the human basicranium. Symposium on Development of the Basicranium. Edited by Bosma, J.F., NIDR; DHEW Public No. (NIH) 77-989, Bethesda, Md., 1977.)

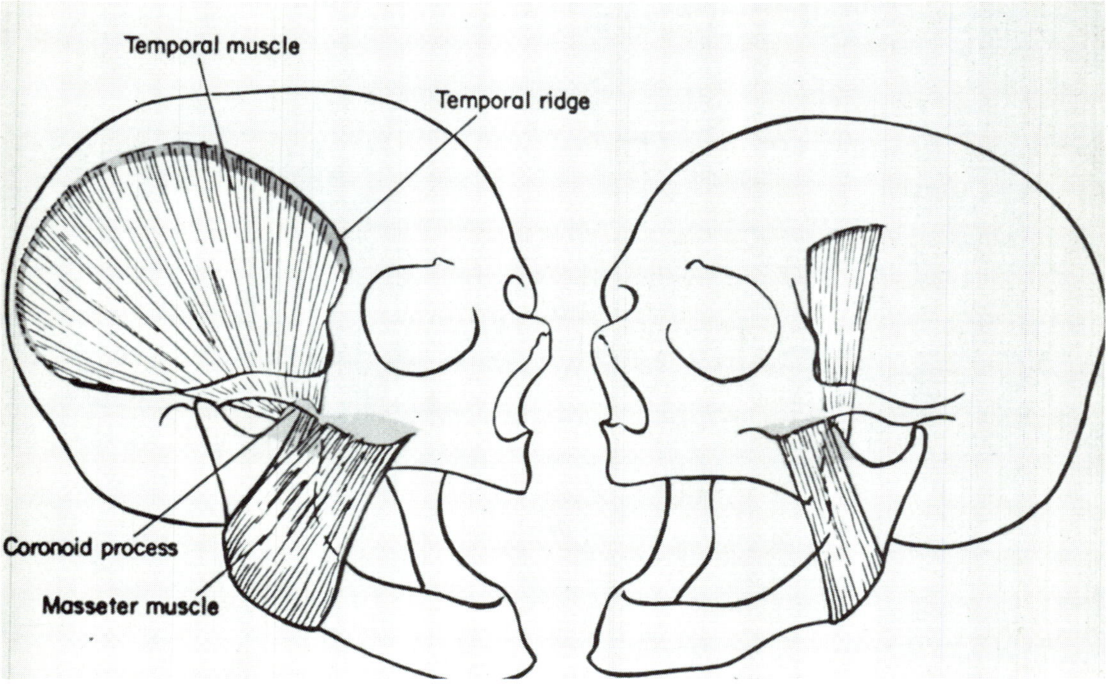

Figure 4–33. Mechanical force relationships between function and form as illustrated in a 60-year-old man who had a unilateral seventh nerve palsy from early in life. On the affected side the facial muscles were quite small, and all the sites of muscle attachment were less prominent on the affected side.

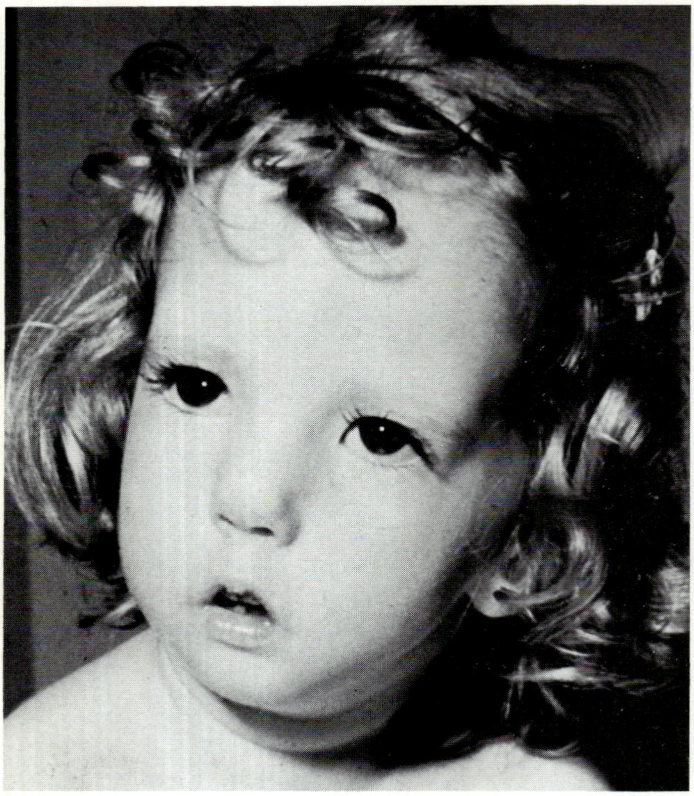

Figure 4–34. This girl is lacking sixth and seventh nerve function, a problem referred to as Moebius malformation sequence. The facial impact is *secondary* to the long standing deficit of forces in the developing face. The almond-shaped eye is interpreted as being secondary to a deficiency of orbicularis oculi function, the small alae nasae to a deficit in the muscles that attach to this cartilage, and the small mouth to a lack of orbicularis oris muscle function. The shallow temporal region is ascribed to weakness of the temporal muscle, the shallow malar region to deficit of masseter function, and the small mandible to a diminished function of the mandible.

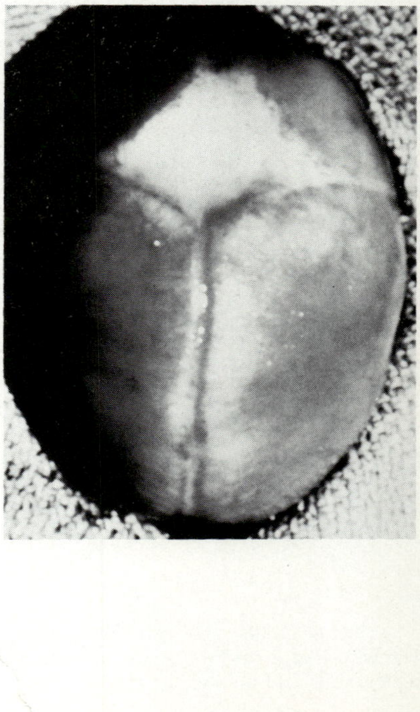

Figure 4–35. The calvarium in a 20 week fetus showing anterior fontanel and sutures.

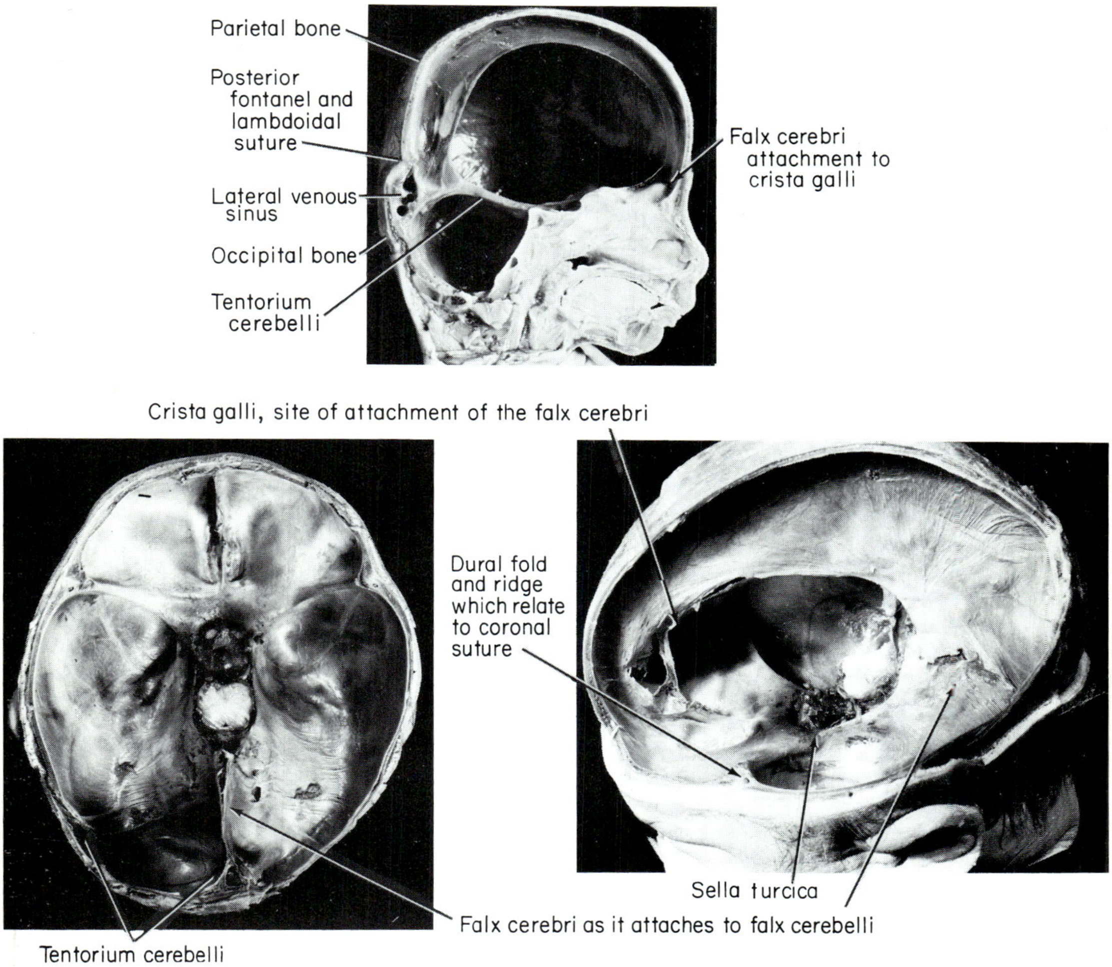

Figure 4–36. The dural reflections, which relate mechanically to the recesses in the developing brain, are shown above at 16 weeks and below in a term baby. Note how the lines of growth stretch are evident in the alignment of collagen fibrils within the dura. (From Professors Töndury and Kubik, University of Zurich.)

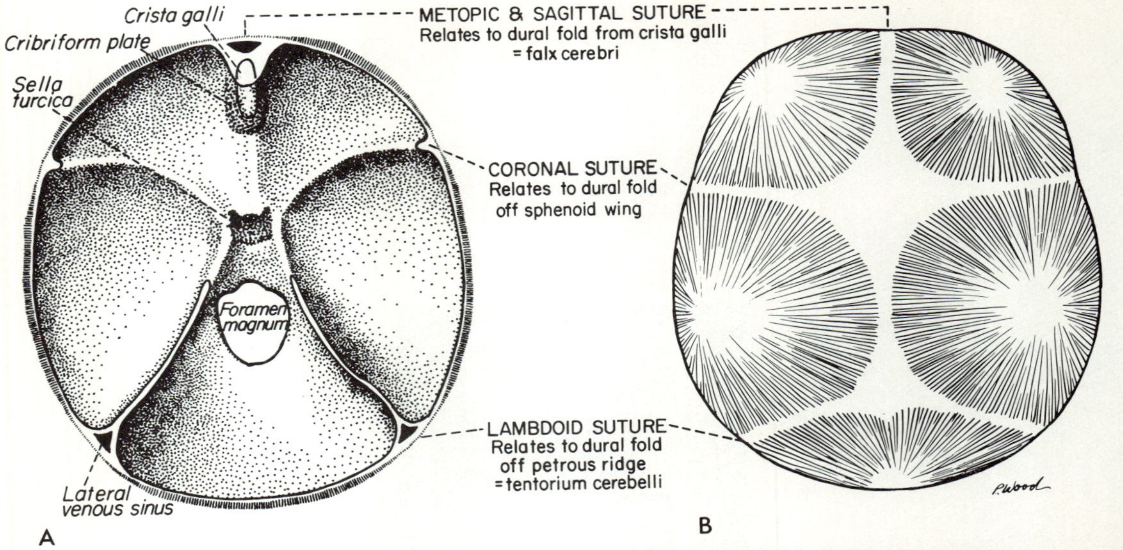

Figure 4–37. Conceptual drawing from a 17 week fetus, by which time the early calvarium is formed. The basilar view (left) shows the sites of dural reflection from the crista galli, sphenoid wings, and petrous ridges. These dural reflections are the sites of passive sutural development, as shown to the right. The top view of the early calvarium shows how ossification begins in the central spots between the dural reflections and spreads centrifugally toward the sutures. (From Smith, D.W., and Töndury, G.: Am. J. Dis. Child. *132*:662, 1978.)

sites of the sutures. The metopic and sagittal sutures relate to the sites of the dural reflection into the interhemispheral fissure, the falx cerebri. The lambdoid sutures relate to the sites of the dural reflection between the cerebrum and cerebellum, the falx cerebelli. The coronal suture relates to the insular sulcus of the brain with its dural reflection off the sphenoid wing, which faithfully fills in this sulcus in the brain.

Between the sites of dural reflection, ossification begins within the membranous dura. These niduses of ossification spread outward toward the sites of the spreading sutures, as shown in Figure 4–37. The radial orientation of the ossification appears to relate to the tensile forces. At the sites of initial ossification in the calvarium there may be small external promontories, most evident in infancy and childhood. These may be noted toward the center of each frontal bone, each parietal bone, and each lateral portion of the occipital bone. They appear to be normal features. The major era in the early development of the calvarium is from 12 to 16 weeks.

In areas of the developing calvarium where the stretch forces may be less concise, such as in the region of the parietal bone near the posterior fontanel, multiple small centers of ossification may develop and then coalesce. These are referred to as wormian bones.

The implication that it is the early brain form that determines the sites of dural reflection and thereby the location of sutures is supported by aberrations of early brain morphogenesis which give rise to altered dural reflections and thereby to variance in the sutures of the calvarium. Examples are shown in Figures 4–38 and 4–39.

There are several means by which the sutures of the calvarium may be altered. These include primary defects of brain, problems in suture development, metabolic problems, and external constraint.

A serious deficit of brain growth, with a lack of stretch at suture lines, whether in primary microcephaly or in a shunted hydrocephalus, may allow for mineralization at one or more of the suture lines. This secondary craniostenosis may then lead to further problems.

A primary defect of brain formation may affect the presence or site of dural reflections and hence the presence and sites of the sutures. One example is holoprosencephaly. A failure of diverticulation of the two cerebral vesicles will yield a single cerebral ventricle and no interhemispheral fissure. This is usually, but not always, accompanied by lack of a metopic suture.

External constraint of the developing fetal head may result in a lack of growth stretch at a given suture and result in craniosynostosis. This appears to be the most common mode of etiology for this problem.

The impact of the craniostenosis on craniofacial form will depend on the age of onset of craniostenosis and the suture(s) involved. Sagittal craniostenosis limits the lateral growth of the calvarium, resulting in a narrow, elongated, sca-

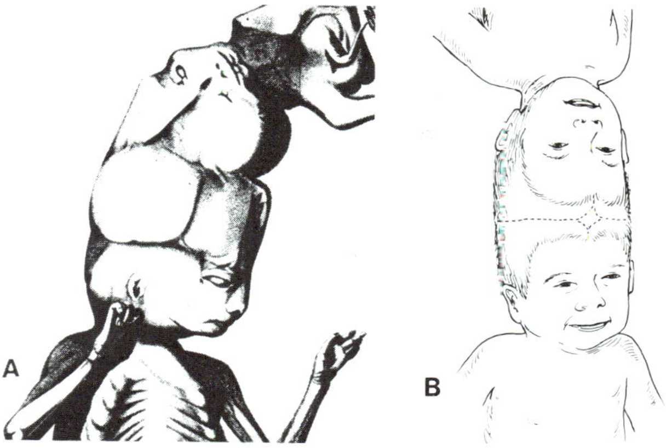

Figure 4–38. Conjoined twins provide an experiment of nature which demonstrates that the suture sites relate to the dural reflections. At the sites of juncture of the two brains there are dural reflections, and at these locations there are sutures and fontanels in positions where they would not normally be present. (From Smith, D.W., and Töndury, G.: Am. J. Dis. Child. *132*: 662, 1978.)

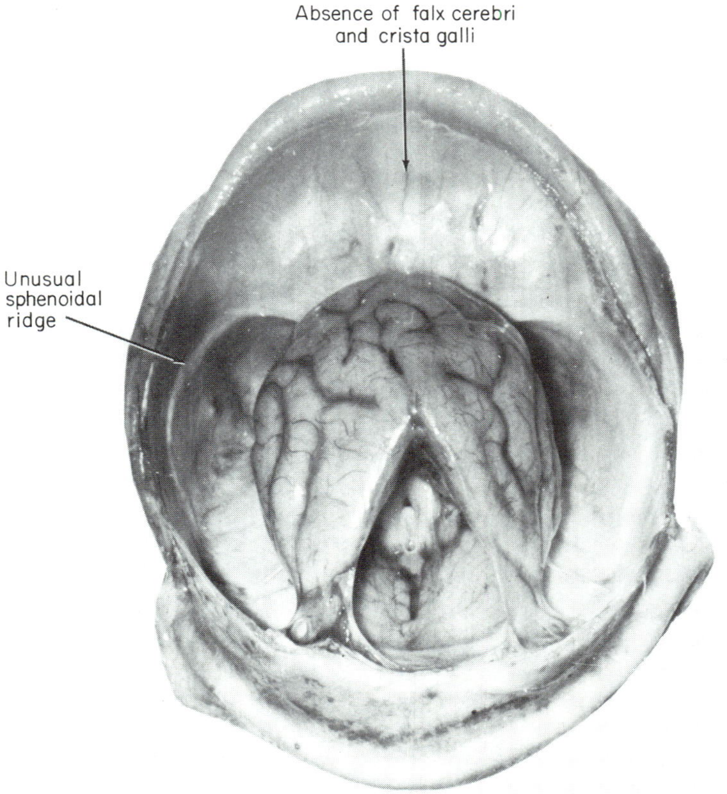

Figure 4–39. An instance of alobar holoprosencephaly. Because there was no interhemispheral fissure, there is no dural reflection at this site (falx cerebri), and as a consequence there is no metopic suture. There is also an aberrant alignment of the sphenoid wings relating to the altered brain impact in this location. This was associated with a comparable aberrant alignment of the coronal sutures. (From DeMeyer, W.: Arch. Neurol. *11*:507, 1964.)

phocephalic head shape. Coronal stenosis limits the anterior-posterior growth, resulting in a short and wide brachycephalic head shape. Early coronal craniostenosis also prevents the forward growth of the brain and hence the anterior growth of the cranial base. Since the cranial base is the roof of the face, the midface tends to be retrusive. Also the orbits become shallow, the eyes more widely spaced, and the forehead high.

Craniostenosis of both the sagittal and coronal sutures will limit the capacity for brain growth and will usually cause increased intracranial pressure. Roentgenograms of the skull may show a beaten-silver appearance. This is at least partially due to a more vertical orientation of the bone fibrils within the calvarium, which tend to align in relation to the altered stress forces. The head tends to become tower-shaped, so-called torencephaly.

The head is quite malleable, especially in fetal life. This is a normal and obviously necessary phenomenon during vaginal delivery. During delivery the bony plates of the calvarium overlap at the sutures, sometimes to a surprising degree. Such molding is usually transient, being limited to a few days.

Prolonged uterine constraint with compression of the fetal head during late fetal life may give rise to deformations of the head which only slowly resolve with time, or which may merit management in achieving a more normal resolution.

The Cranial Base. The anterior cranial base develops from cartilage that becomes ossified, with persisting epiphysis-like growth centers posterior and anterior to the sella turcica. The region from the sella turcica anteriorly, which is designated as the anterior cranial base, tends to grow forward in accordance with frontal brain growth. Hence, its growth follows that of neural growth, with 56 per cent completed by birth and 70 per cent completed by the age of two years.[12] It is important to appreciate that the anterior cranial base is the roof of the face from which the maxillary-ethmoid complex projects downward and the anterior portion is the nasal bridge, as shown in Figure 4–31.

A deficit of frontal brain growth may yield a shorter cranial base and a less prominent nasal bridge. A shorter cranial base will generally yield a flatter facial profile with a tendency toward a smaller and retrusive mid-face.

Eyes. The early outpouchings from the diencephalon, the optic cups, induce the formation of a lens in the overlying ectoderm: thus begins the formation of the eye. Surrounding mesenchymal cells condense to form the globular eye capsule within which the collagen fibrils align in relationship to the fluid pressure from within the eye. Around the eye the mesenchymal tissues condense to form the bony orbit, which conforms to and is shaped in relation to the eye.[11]

A problem of fluid mechanics within the eye may result in increased pressure (glaucoma). This tends to distort the shape of the tense eye toward greater anterior globular prominence. It may also result in cloudiness of the cornea and destructive changes within the eye leading to eventual blindness.

A small eye (microphthalmia) will yield a small orbit. A lack of any optic cup will yield *no* orbit.[11] The accessory tissues of muscles, lacrimal apparatus, eyebrows, eyelids, and eyelashes all relate to the development of the early optic evagination.[11] For example, an altered position of the early orbit is accompanied by predictable secondary development of all these accessory structures in the aberrant position of the optic vesicle, as exemplified in Figure 4–40.

Ears. *Inner Ear*: The otic placode, which is neural type tissue, invaginates from the surface ectoderm to become the otocyst. The differential growth of the otocyst leads to the beautiful spiral of the cochlea and the form of the vestibular apparatus. The mesenchyme around the otic placode is induced to form cartilage which faithfully conforms in its shape and which exerts a major role in the development of the sphenoid wing.

Middle Ear: The derivatives of the second and third brachial arches form the malleus, incus, and stapes as a connecting functional link between the eardrum and the round window of

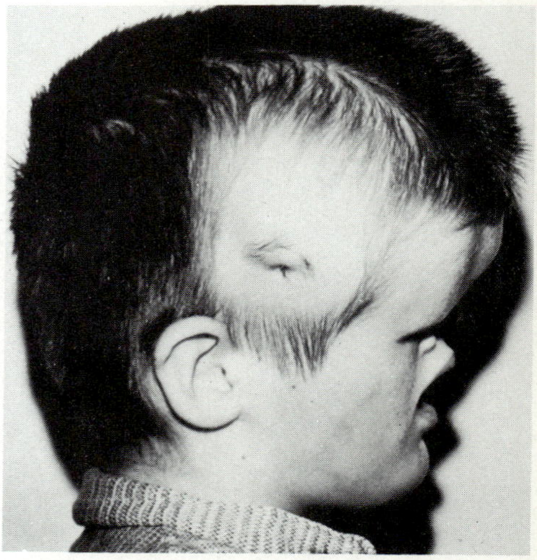

Figure 4–40. A rudimentary eye projected to an unusual temporal location in this individual. At this site the early optic vesicle mechanically gave rise to the development of a small optic cup. Furthermore, there was the development of periocular muscles, lacrimal apparatus, and eyelids, plus the growth of the hair at the eyebrow location and a zone of periocular hair growth suppression. (From Smith, D.W., and Gong, B.T.: Teratology 9:17, 1974.)

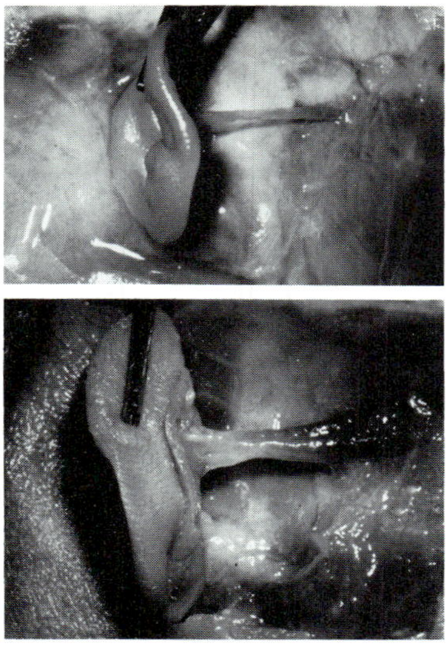

Figure 4–41. The posterior auricular muscle attaches from the concha of the ear to the mastoid region, thus holding the auricle toward the head. The upper photo is from a 16 week fetus and the lower a 20 week fetus. (From Smith, D.W., and Takashima, H.: Lancet *1*:747, 1978.)

the cochlea, thus transmitting the vibrations to the cochlea. Any ankylosis within the joints of these bones may result in a problem of conductive deafness.

External Ear: The external auricle forms from the cartilaginous cores of the early hillocks of Hiss, which blend into a sheet of cartilage that grows throughout life. Mild to moderate deformations of the external auricle are common in the newly born baby, relating to constraint of the pliable auricle in late fetal life. Oligohydramnios accentuates such deformation and may result in an "accordioned" ear, an ear that is flattened against the calvarium, or other changes. The shoulder may be pressed up under the auricle in such situations as breech presentation and result in uplifting of the lower auricle. These distortions tend to resolve toward normal form after birth and are thoroughly benign deformations.

A distended jugular lymph sac, such as frequently occurs in the XO Turner fetus, may distort the auricle, making it more prominent and slanted than usual.

The position and form of the cartilaginous folds of the auricle relate largely to the sites of insertion and origin of the auricular muscles.[14] Thus, defects of form of the external auricle may be the consequence of aberration in development and/or function of particular ear muscles. For example, absence of the posterior auricular ear muscle, which normally holds the ear in toward the calvarium, results in a protruding auricle (see Figs. 4–41 and 4–42), while absence of the superior auricular ear muscle results in a folded-over "lop" ear which may appear low in place-

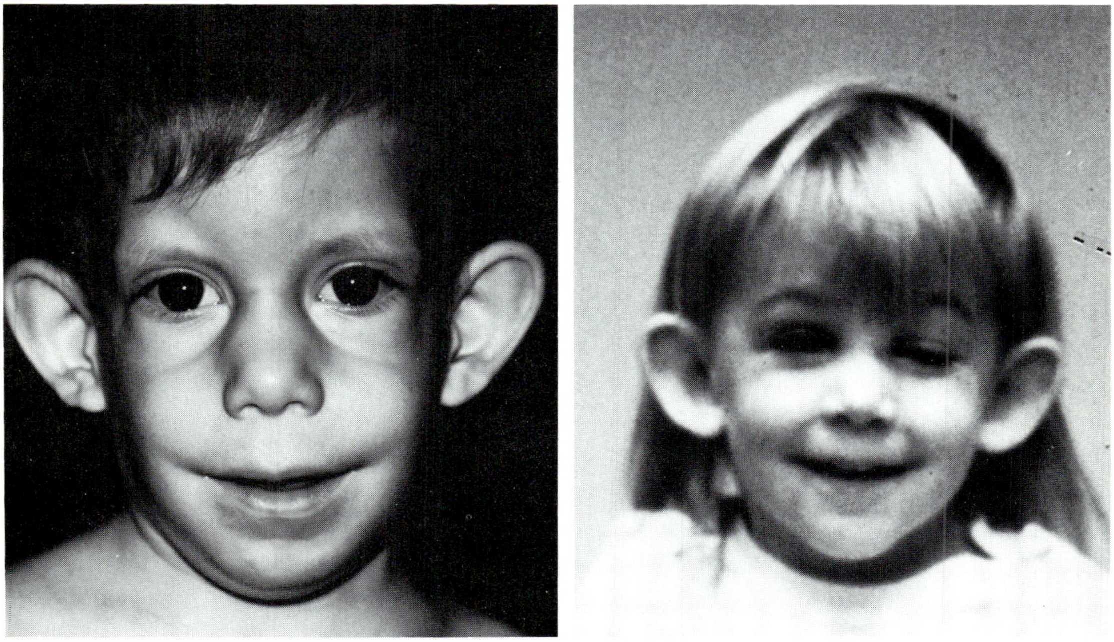

Figure 4–42. *Left,* a boy with neuromuscular weakness who had protruding ears as one feature. *Right,* a girl with XO Turner syndrome who has protruding ears plus unilateral ptosis of the eyelid. The protruding ears are a secondary mechanical neuromuscular sign, as is the ptosis of the eyelid. For each, the question is raised whether the primary problem is neurological or muscular. (From Smith, D.W., and Takashima, H.: Lancet *1*:747, 1978.)

ment (see Figs. 4–43 and 4–44). The inner conchal plical folds appear to relate to the intrinsic auricular ear muscles, and defects in their development may result in varying degrees of a simple form to the concha. Experimental studies in the rodent have shown that early denervation of the seventh nerve, which supplies the auricular ear muscles, will result in a simple auricle that lacks the usual conchal folds.

Nose and Nasopharynx. The neural olfactory pit invaginates from the surface ectoderm and then sends its axons to synapse with those of the olfactory lobes. Later, when the base of the skull becomes cartilage and bone, these axons create the sites of "perforation" in the cribriform plate. Around the edges of the olfactory pit, the median and lateral nasal swellings rapidly grow out and coalesce with the maxillary swelling, to form much of the external nose and to fuse inferiorly to form the upper lip. The invaginating olfactory

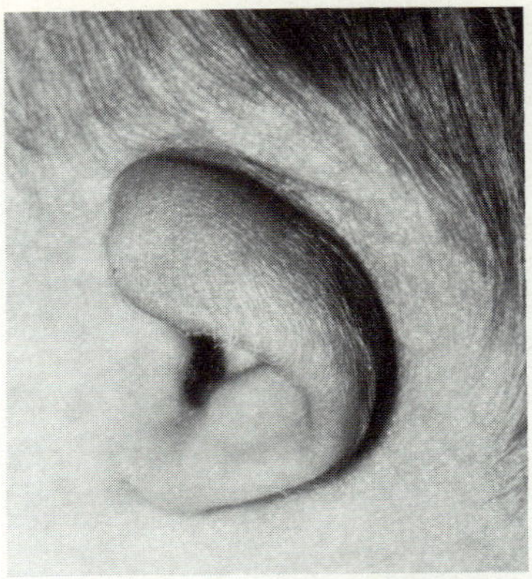

Figure 4–43. Lop ear, a secondary deformation due to a defect in development of function of the superior auricular ear muscle, which attaches the superior auricle to the head.

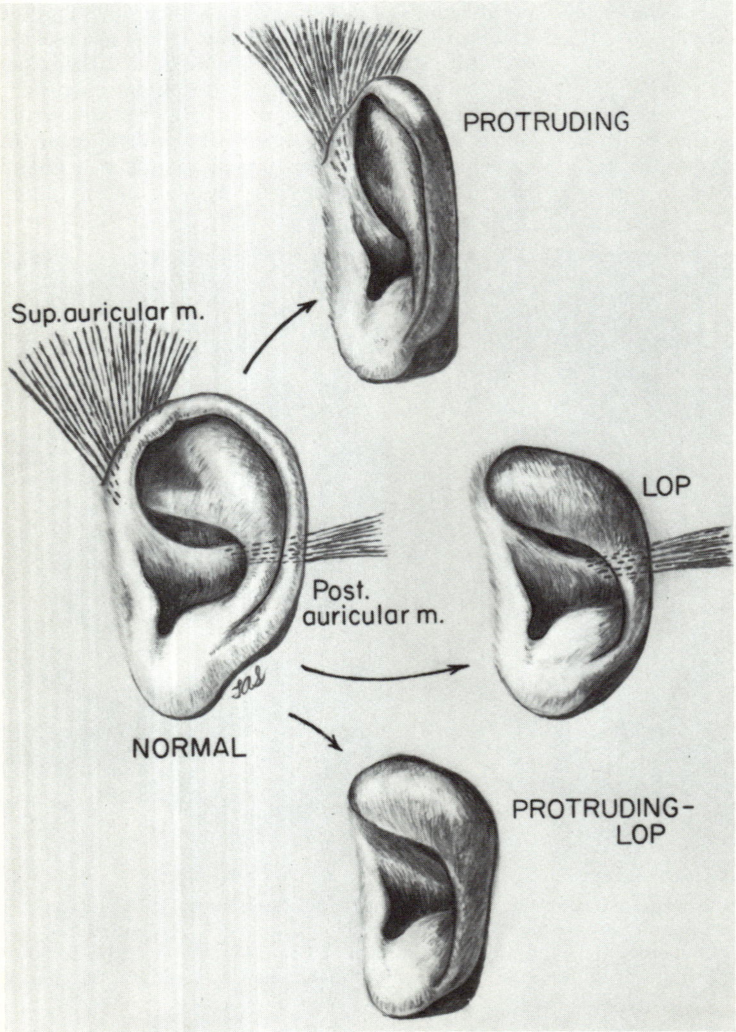

Figure 4–44. Summary of relationship between the extrinsic ear muscles and ear form. (Courtesy of Thomas Stebbins, University of Washington School of Medicine.)

pits meet posteriorly with the foregut, and the epithelium between them breaks down, providing ready communication between the nasal and oral cavities. The cartilaginous nasal septum is in direct continuity with the anterior base of the skull, and hence alterations in growth of the base of the skull may secondarily affect the nasal situation. Fusion of the maxillary palatine shelves with the nasal septum separates the nasal cavity from the mouth proper. Cartilaginous plates develop in the ala nasi, and these have muscle attachments that allow for constriction of the nares. Within the nose the cartilaginous turbinates grow, and evaginations from the nasal cavity occur into the surrounding bone. These evaginations, the sinuses, aerate the surrounding bones. This substantially reduces their weight while still providing excellent structural support. Sinus development is largely incomplete at birth. The first pharyngeal pouch persists as the eustachian tube and middle ear. Evaginations from the middle ear aerate the mastoid portion of the temporal bone, in similar fashion to the sinuses.

Late uterine constraint may distort the nose. Most commonly it may be compressed to one side. After birth this usually resolves spontaneously, though some manual pulling and remolding may be merited. Persisting compression may limit the growth of the nose, as in a face presentation. However, postnatal catch-up growth will usually result in a restoration to normal form.

As previously mentioned, aberrations of the growth of the cranial base, such as with problems of frontal brain growth, may alter both the relative position of the nasal bridge and the position and form of the nose.

Problems with the development and/or function of the musculature of the ala nasi may result in a narrow nose with small alar wings.

The sinuses tend to extend well into the solid bone that surrounds them. If there is a loss of permanent teeth from the upper jaw, the maxillary sinus will extend further than usual, coming into close proximity with the alveolar ridge at the sites of the missing teeth.

Palate and Tongue. The palatal shelves, which are initially projecting downward alongside the tongue, undergo a shift into the horizontal position and then fuse from front to back with each other and with the nasal septum. If the mandible is unusually small, there may be posterior displacement of the tongue which will tend to occlude closure of the palatal shelves, giving rise to a U-shaped palatal defect,[15] as shown in Figures 4–45 through 4–47. The posteriorly displaced tongue may obstruct the posterior pharynx, giving rise to partial upper airway obstruction at birth. The initiating problem in mandibular size may be a malformation, and

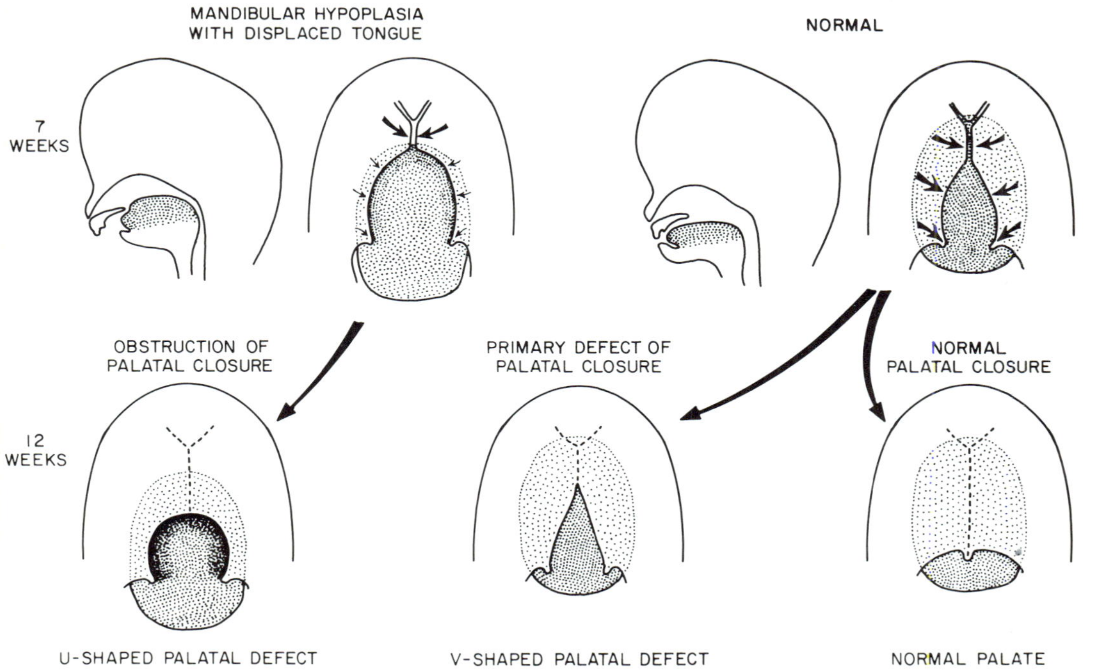

Figure 4–45. Pathways leading to defects of palatal closure as viewed in the lateral aspect and from above the palate. The left side shows lingual obstruction to closure of normal palatine shelves because of a small mandible with retroplaced tongue. This leads to a U-shaped palatal defect. The right side shows the normal closure of the palatine shelves and the V-shaped palatine defect which results from a primary problem in their closure. (From Hanson, J.W., and Smith, D.W.: J. Pediat. *87*:30, 1975.)

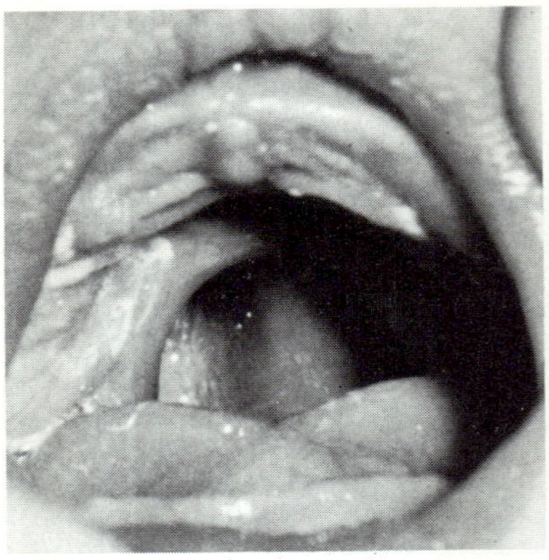

Figure 4–46. Robin sequence with U-shaped palatal defect secondary to interposition of the retroplaced tongue, itself the consequence of a small mandible. Note that the retroplaced tongue has allowed the development of prominent rugous ridging in the anterior portion of the palate. (From Hanson, J.W., and Smith, D.W.: J. Pediatr. *87*:30, 1975.)

hence the consequences are termed the early micrognathia malformation sequence, or the Robin malformation sequence. The small mandible might also be the result of early fetal constraint with limitation of mandibular growth; in this instance the diagnosis would tend toward early micrognathia *deformation* sequence.

Not only does the tongue play a significant mechanical role in palatine closure but it also exerts a major impact on palatal form. Normally there are lateral palatine ridges that extend down from the roof of the palate between the alveolar ridges and the central palate, as shown in Figure 4–48.[16] These ridges are prominent in fetal life and are composed of mucopolysaccharide-rich connective tissue and myriads of small salivary glands. The force of the tongue thrust tends to smooth them out during fetal life.

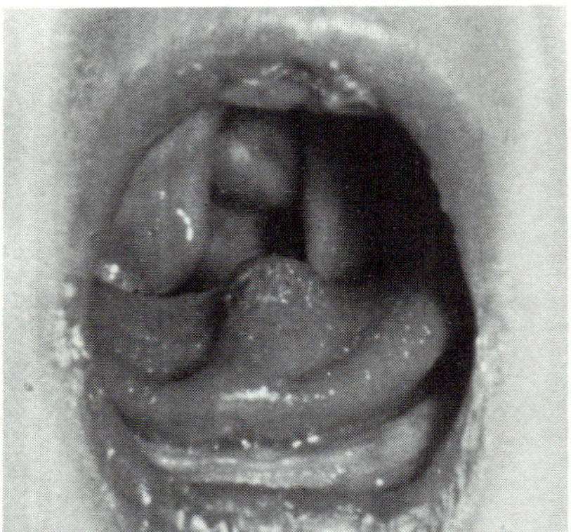

Figure 4–47. U-shaped palatal defect with molding of the tongue, which apparently remained partially interposed between the palatal shelves from early in development.

Any disorder that limits tongue thrust into the palate, such as hypotonia, other neurological deficits, or microglossia, will cause prominent lateral palatine ridges (see Fig. 4–48), often giving the appearance of a "narrow, high-arched" palate. At the other extreme, an enlarged tongue may result in relative flattening and even broadening of the hard palate. Thus the tongue, a very strong muscle, exerts a major impact within the mouth.

A narrow palate that appears highly arched not uncommonly develops in children with mental deficiency (see Fig. 4–49). The reason for this is not clear. I would suspect that it most likely relates to a deficit in functional usage of the facial musculature. A narrow palate may also develop in patients with coronal suture craniostenosis.

Alveolar Ridge, Teeth, and Mandible. The tooth anlagen develop as ectodermal downgrowths that interact with the underlying mesenchyme to form the teeth, which then erupt, usually through the channel of their original downgrowth. If there is a failure of tooth development the alveolar ridge lacks prominence at that region. Thus the major mass of the alveolar ridges relates to the teeth. The form of the enamel crown of a tooth, which is produced by the ectodermal component, is genetically determined and allows for amazing interdigitation between the upper and lower teeth. The forces of biting and chewing tend to foster alignment of the teeth. The growth of the lower jaw — the mandible — tends to follow the lead of the upper jaw. This applies to lateral growth as well. Thus, if the maxilla is narrow, the mandible will also tend to be narrow. However, a deficit of function of the mandible will tend to slow its growth rate.

The muscles of the mandible are powerful and their sites of attachment give rise to bony promontories. Figure 4–33 shows the impact of a unilateral facial nerve palsy on these muscles and therefore on the bony form of the face. The impact of the facial muscles on bony promontories is dramatically exemplified by experimental studies in rodents. For example, early resection of the masseter muscle results in a complete lack of the coronoid process, its site of insertion on the mandible (Fig. 4–50).

If the teeth are crowded, one or more may erupt in an aberrant alignment. Usually the easiest management is removal of the tooth that is "crowded out." Malalignment of the teeth is not uncommon. Orthodontic methods of constraint have become a common practice in realignment of the teeth and jaws during childhood.

Thorax and Lung. The growth of the ribs and the thoracic cage is integral to the full development of the lungs. The lungs develop as a progressive arborization from an outbudding of the foregut. The septation of the thoracic and abdominal cavities by the diaphragm allows the fetus to make respiratory movements. The full growth of the thoracic cage is important during

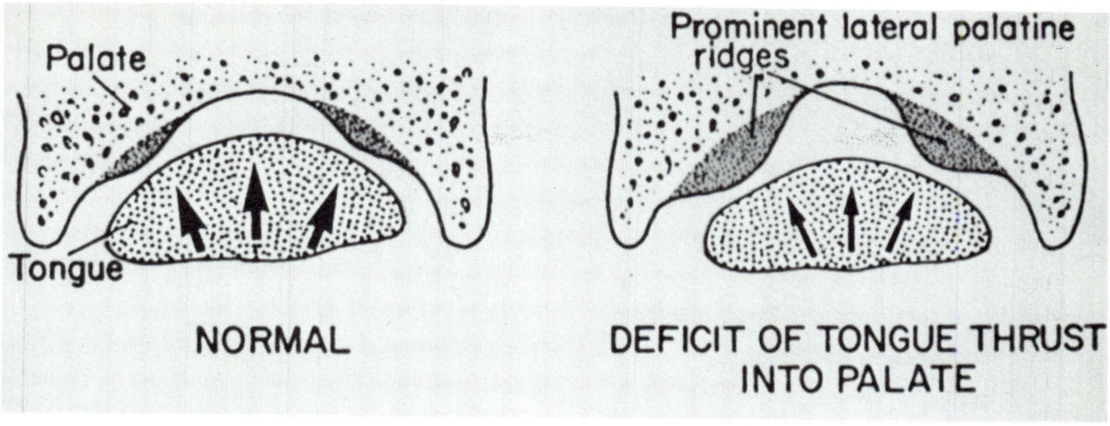

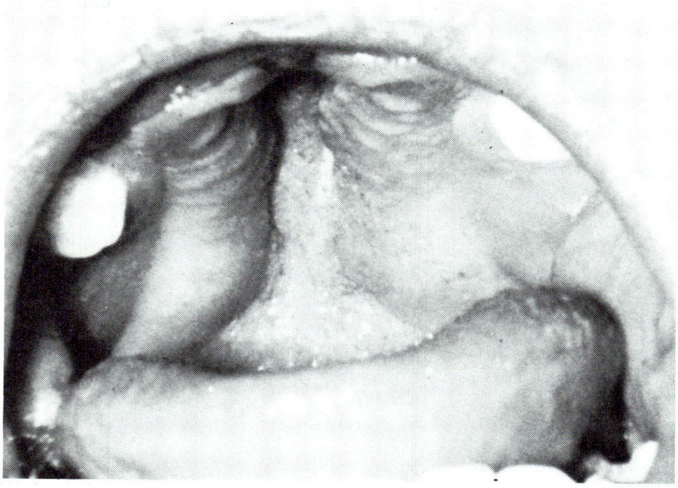

Figure 4–48. *Above,* cross section depiction of palate and tongue in a normal infant and one in whom there was a deficit of tongue thrust into the hard palate, which allowed for the development of prominent lateral palatal ridges. *Below,* prominent lateral palatine shelves between the alveolar ridges and the center of the palate in this hypotonic infant indicated that the hypotonia was of long standing.

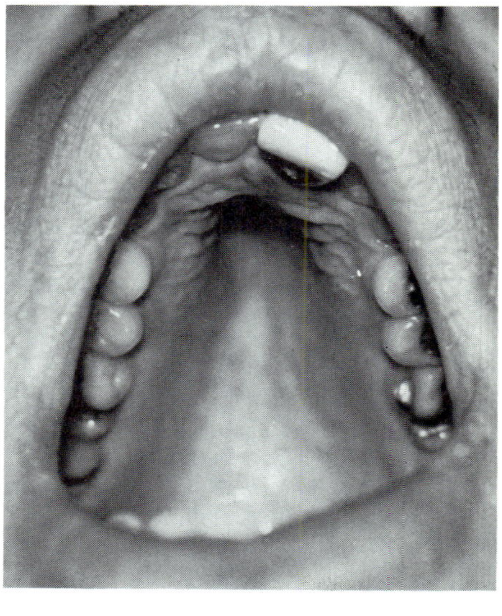

Figure 4–49. Narrow palate in a mentally retarded adult, the presumed consequences of the deficiency of normal forces relative to the growth and form of the maxilla. Such a narrow palate is unusual in mentally retarded infants but not in retarded older children.

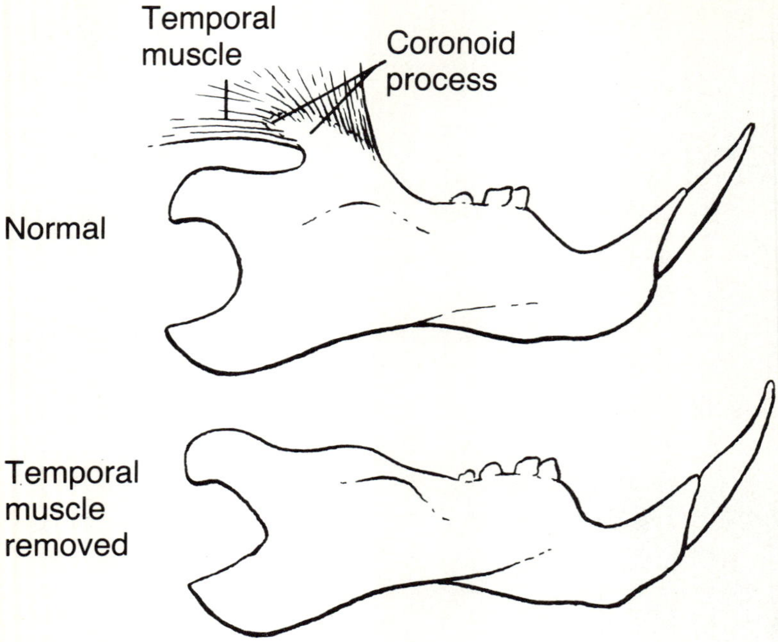

Figure 4–50. Early postnatal removal of the masseter muscle in the rat results in a lack of the coronoid process of the mandible, the bony protuberance that normally results from the tension of the masseter muscle at this site of attachment.

the latter phase of lung development when the lung progresses from a solid organ tissue to one with alveolar sacs capable of aeration. Restrictive crowding during the late fetal lung growth may result in the lung being incompletely developed by birth, and the infant will have respiratory insufficiency and may develop the pathological consequences termed hyaline membrane disease. Deficit of lung growth may be due to a number of causes, as summarized in Table 4–3. External constraint of an unusual degree, such as a bicornuate uterus, may be a cause. With oligohydramnios, the constraint to thoracic growth is frequently sufficient to impair full lung development.[17] As a consequence, respiratory insufficiency is the predominant cause of death in newborn babies affected by oligohydramnios. Crowding of the lung during growth may be intrinsic, as in diaphragmatic hernia. A diaphragmatic "hernia," of course, represents incomplete development of the diaphragm. This allows variable amounts of abdominal contents to gain access to the thoracic cage and limits the capacity for full lung growth. Hence, the newly born baby with a diaphragmatic hernia usually dies of respiratory insufficiency, even if an excellent diaphragmatic repair with removal of abdominal contents from the thoracic cage is done soon after birth.

The thoracic cage is rather malleable and may show alterations of form in relation to constraint. If the fetus is in a position with the chin forced into the chest, for example, there may be both a small mandible and a mild "impression" on the chest wall.

Cardiovascular. The early heart ducts fuse to become one tube which then undergoes almost a figure eight type of contortion to become the four-chambered heart. Growth of specific ridges within the convoluting heart-to-be gives rise to separation of the blood channels and develop-

Table 4–3. Causes of Inadequate Late Fetal Lung Growth

	GENERAL	EXAMPLES
EXTERNAL CONSTRAINT	Oligohydramnios	Renal agenesis Chronic leakage of amniotic fluid
	Small uterine cavity	Bicornuate uterus Large uterine fibroid(s)
INTRINSIC CONSTRAINT	Limited thoracic growth	Thoracic asphyxiant dystrophy
	Thoracic mass	Diaphragmatic hernia

ment of the valves. Thus, the growth of the atrioventricular cushions assists in the separation of the atria and ventricles and the formation of the tricuspid and mitral valves, whereas the growth of the conotruncal pads separates the single outlet truncus into the aorta and pulmonary arteries with the development of aortic and pulmonary valves. Throughout cardiac morphogenesis the direction and force of the streams of blood play a major role in the development of cardiac form. For example, the blood coming from the placenta through the ductus venosus flows across the right atrium and maintains the patency of the foramen ovale, directly shunting the blood into the left atrium. As soon as the large placental flow ceases at birth and other changes take place, such as closure of the ductus arteriosus and the "opening up" of the pulmonary vascular bed, the direction and magnitude of blood flow change in such a manner as to close the foramen ovale.

Any anatomical change in early heart development will usually have a major effect on subsequent cardiac morphogenesis, by having changed the biomechanics within the developing heart. For example, a ventricular septal defect will result in excessive shunting of blood into the right ventricle and the pulmonary system, thus resulting in enlargement of the right ventricle. The excessive pressure on the pulmonary circulation will eventually cause increased vascular resistance, further increasing the load on the right ventricle, which may then begin to fail in its function. Early intervention, with closure of the ventricular septal defect, may prevent such biomechanical consequences, all of which may be interpreted as *deformations* in the cardiovascular system.

Interference with the early flow patterns may be the primary cause of problems in cardiac morphogenesis. Ishikawa[18] produced defects of the heart and great vessels in 42 per cent of chick embryos by placing them in a centrifuge for nine hours during the period of cardiac morphogenesis. The cardiac defects were presumed to be the consequence of the alterations in the flow patterns during this critical time in heart development.

The peripheral blood vessels develop as a coalescence of multiple small lacunae into vessels. Initially there tends to be a general network of small vessels. The magnitude and direction of flow will result in enlargement of some of these minute vessels in a particular direction, whereas a diminished flow will result in regression of vessels. Hence the vascularity develops to a major extent in relation to the needs of the region and to its form. If there is hypoplasia in a region, the vascular channels in that region will generally be smaller than usual.

Intestines. The endoderm outpouches in a forward direction as the foregut and posteriorly as the hindgut. As the intestine enlarges it extends beyond the abdominal wall into the allantoic sac and then returns later into the abdominal cavity. Its enlargement gives rise to multiple foldings in the gut and to overall rotation of the midgut so that the cecum ends up in the right lower quadrant. The capsule of the intestine — the peritoneum — follows this rotation and then becomes fixed to the inner abdominal wall at certain points. An incomplete rotation of the gut will result in unusual mesenteric attachments and will increase the liability toward volvulus of the midgut.

Any obstruction of the intestine will alter mechanics within the gut, giving rise to distention of the proximal gut and changes in the bowel wall. The distal segment, with less distention, will be unusually small in caliber.

Urinary Tract and Kidneys. The early mesonephric ridge has a longitudinal series of nephron elements that drain into a common mesonephric duct. Toward the lower end of this duct an outpouching occurs — the ureteral bud. This induces the formation of glomeruli and nephron elements in the adjacent metanephric blastema. The ureteral bud progressively arborizes, and each new bud induces a new group of glomeruli and nephrons, which communicate with the ureteral buds. The ureteral bud becomes the ureter, and its multiple branches become the collecting ducts and distal tubules. The induced elements become the glomeruli and the proximal renal tubules. If there is any obstruction to the flow of urine, which begins by eight to nine weeks in the human, the area proximal to the obstruction will become dilated. If the flow from a whole kidney is obstructed the pelvic drainage system of the kidney becomes dilated; this is termed hydronephrosis. If it occurs during early development it may adversely affect renal morphogenesis in such a manner as to result in hypoplasia and the formation of "cysts" in the kidney. These are not true cysts, rather they are dilations in the tubules that may appear as cysts on histological sections of the kidney.

Early obstruction to urine flow in the urethra results in the urethral obstruction malformation sequence, a series of consequences of the biomechanical effects of obstruction within the urinary tract.[19]

Any renal system disorder that results in a lack of urine flow into the amniotic space will usually cause a deficit of amniotic fluid during late fetal life. It does not matter whether the lack of urine is due to renal agenesis or to severe urethral obstruction, the consequences are the same — the oligohydramnios deformation sequence.

REFERENCES

1. Thompson, D.: On Growth and Form. A New Edition. Cambridge, The University Press, 1942.
2. Dunn, P.M.: Growth retardation of infants with

congenital postural deformities. Acta Med. Auxol. *7*:63, 1975.
3. Hafez, E.S.E.: *In* Benirschke, K.: Comparative Aspects of Reproductive Failure. New York, Springer-Verlag, 1967.
4. Smith, G.E.: The causation of the symmetrical thinning of the parietal bones in ancient Egyptians. J. Anat. Physiol. London *41*:232, 1906–7.
5. Drachman, D.B., and Coulombre, A. J.: Experimental clubfoot and arthrogryposis multiplex congenita. Lancet *2*:523, 1962.
6. Jago, R.H.: Arthrogryposis following treatment of maternal tetanus with muscle relaxants. Arch. Dis. Child. *45*:277, 1970.
7. Smith, D.W.: Redundant skin folds in the infant; their origin and relevance. J. Pediatr. *94*:1021, 1979.
8. Smith, D.W., and Gong, B.T.: Scalp hair patterning as a clue to early fetal brain development. J. Pediatr. *83*:374, 1973.
9. Mulvihill, J.J., and Smith, D.W.: Genesis of dermatoglyphics. J. Pediatr. *75*:579, 1969.
10. Popich, G.A., and Smith, D.W.: The genesis and significance of digital and palmar hand creases: Preliminary report. J. Pediatr. *77*:1017, 1960.
11. Jones, K.L., Higginbottom, M.C., and Smith, D.W.: The determining role of the optic vesicles in orbital and periocular development and placement. Pediatr. Res. *14*:703, 1980.
12. Smith, D.W., and Töndury, G.: Origin of the calvaria and its sutures. Am. J. Dis. Child. *132*:662, 1978.
13. Graham, J.M., deSaxe, M., and Smith, D.W.: Sagittal craniostenosis: Fetal head constraint as one possible cause. J. Pediatr. *95*:747, 1979.
14. Smith, D.W., and Takashima, H.: Protruding auricle: A neuromuscular sign. Lancet *1*:747, 1978.
15. Hanson, J.W., and Smith, D.W.: U-shaped palatal defect in the Robin anomalad: Developmental and clinical relevance. J. Pediatr. *87*:30, 1975.
16. Hanson, J.W., Smith, D.W., and Cohen, M.M., Jr: Prominent lateral palatine ridges: Developmental and clinical relevance. J. Pediatr. *89*:54, 1976.
17. Thomas, I.T., and Smith, D.W.: Oligohydramnios, cause of the non-renal features of Potter's syndrome, including pulmonary hypoplasia. J. Pediatr. *84*:811, 1974.
18. Ishikawa, Prof., Tokyo University Medical School. Personal communication.
19. Pagon, R.A., Smith, D.W., and Shepard, T.H.: Urethral obstruction malformation complex: A cause of abdominal muscle deficiency and the "prune belly." J. Pediatr. *96*:900, 1979.

Chapter Five

CONCLUDING REMARKS

Ever since Peter Dunn acquainted me with the basic concepts of deformation I have been increasingly impressed by the frequency with which unusual mechanical forces may be deduced as being responsible for structural birth defects. The impact of mechanical forces on form not only has provided an understanding of the extrinsic constraint deformations but also has led to the appreciation that many of the malformation sequences can be interpreted as an initiating malformation that gave rise to altered mechanical forces and a cascade of intrinsic deformation. Furthermore, this mechanical perspective provides a better understanding of factors in normal morphogenesis.

The major emphasis of this text has been on the extrinsic constraint deformations that are secondary to crowding in utero. These should, to the extent possible, be distinguished from malformations with or without secondary intrinsic deformation. Not only are there major differences in the etiology, prognosis, management, and recurrence risk counsel but there also is a profound difference in the attitude that can be conveyed to the parents. The child with extrinsic deformation may usually be interpreted as normal, and the parents can look forward to the restoration of normal form. This attitude toward considering the extrinsic deformations as a separable category of birth defects is also critical toward providing better answers relative to etiology and prevention. The etiological factors that may cause extrinsic deformation are obviously very different from those that cause malformation problems. The preventive measures for extrinsic deformations are also different and entail such considerations as the controversial external version for malposition in utero and the surgical reconstruction of a malformed uterus. Furthermore, since extrinsic deformations are more common in infants of primigravida mothers and in the larger fetuses, it is quite reasonable to anticipate that the incidence of extrinsic deformations might increase as a consequence of smaller families and larger babies.

The basic principles of extrinsic deformation are simple. The magnitude and direction of force have their impact on form. The same simple precepts are relevant to the reformational management. With rare exception this may be accomplished by rational application of subtle forces.

Why has it taken such a long time for this knowledge to become an integral part of medicine? It is not because extrinsic deformations are rare — they are common. It is not because the concepts are new — they are old. Possibly one reason is that the overall concepts that relate to the developmental pathology, diagnosis, and management of extrinsic deformations are so simple. In recent times there has been a tendency to look for more complex answers of a biochemical and physiologic nature and to bypass the simple mechanistic approaches. Hence this book is dedicated to bringing the mechanical aspects of morphogenesis and deformation into the mainstream of medicine, where they belong.

Very few studies of extrinsic deformation in experimental animals have been done. One reason is that few creatures other than man tend to outgrow the uterus prior to birth and to have constraint deformations at birth. This is one price the slowly aging, rapidly growing, large-brained human must pay for his or her present level of evolvement.

Index

Note: Page numbers in *italic* type refer to illustrations; page numbers followed by (t) refer to tables.